'I started reading this book in the garden on a lovely spring evening. I was gripped immediately. Suddenly I was transported to Catherine Jessop's Christmas 2016, when her husband's life and that of her whole family was thrown into disarray by a dreadful illness I know only too well. Although I have studied the terrible brain inflammation, encephalitis, for 25 years, and met thousands of patients, I learnt a lot from this compelling narrative, about fear, hope, survival, endurance and, above all, love.'

– Professor Tom Solomon, Professor of Neurology at the University of Liverpool and President of the Encephalitis Society

'When illness enters the life of a family, things rarely remain the same. Catherine Jessop's poignant and searingly honest account of how her family's life was thrown off course in the wake of her husband's diagnosis of encephalitis provides a wealth of essential practical information and tips for coping. It is a beacon of hope for others facing the rollercoaster ride of life-changing illness – read and be guided by its wisdom.'

– Dr Audrey Daisley, Consultant Clinical Neuropsychologist, Oxford

'Encephalitis is a thief! The Jessop family know only too well the stealth with which it approaches, the immediacy with which it strikes and the devastation it leaves in its wake. In *Pulling Through* they use their journey and experience to produce a bible from bedside to the return home, for anyone who finds themselves affected by sudden-onset ill-health in their family.'

– Dr Ava Easton, Chief Executive, Encephalitis Society

PULLING THROUGH

of related interest

The Patient Revolution
How We Can Heal the Healthcare System
David Gilbert
ISBN 978 1 78592 538 2
eISBN 978 1 78450 932 3

PULLING THROUGH

Help for Families Navigating Life-Changing Illness

CATHERINE JESSOP

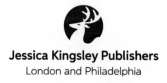

Jessica Kingsley Publishers
London and Philadelphia

First published in Great Britain in 2021 by Jessica Kingsley Publishers
An Hachette Company

1

A CIP catalogue record for this title is available from the
British Library and the Library of Congress

ISBN 978 1 78775 372 3
eISBN 978 1 78775 373 0

Printed and bound in Great Britain by TJ Books Limited

Jessica Kingsley Publishers' policy is to use papers that are natural,
renewable and recyclable products and made from wood grown in
sustainable forests. The logging and manufacturing processes are expected
to conform to the environmental regulations of the country of origin.

Jessica Kingsley Publishers
Carmelite House
50 Victoria Embankment
London EC4Y 0DZ

www.jkp.com

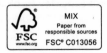

To Izzy, Madeleine and Sam – you are the sunshine of my life.

And to my mum, Clare Fardell (1938–2020), who taught me everything I know about optimism.

CONTENTS

ACKNOWLEDGEMENTS

Thank you so much to the doctors, nurses, RMNs, OTs and all the staff on the hospital ward who worked so tirelessly and with such good humour and patience. In particular, Alan's neurology consultant, who continues to be a calm and reassuring presence in our lives. We are also indebted to all the anonymous scientists, striving to develop ever-better tests and medicines. Without your skill, Alan would not be here.

Thank you to my enormous family. You aren't all mentioned by name in the book, but I can honestly say that every single one of you has made a difference. The same goes for my lovely friends; I am so grateful for your buoyant support and fun.

Three charities have been a tremendous help: Integrated Neurological Services, The Encephalitis Society and Headway. Your work really does improve the lives of those affected by brain injuries.

And finally, a heartfelt thank you to everyone at Jessica Kingsley Publishers – especially Steve, Emma, Vicki and Mark – for all of their encouragement and expertise.

INTRODUCTION

Every year, millions of people in the UK are admitted to hospital for myriad reasons. Most of them are dosed up, patched up or sewn up and sent back home again to carry on much as before. But for some, the trip into hospital marks the moment when an old life ends and a new one begins. That's how it was for us.

We were a family of five, living in the leafy suburbs of a large city. Alan ran his own publishing business and I worked from home. Izzy (20) was in her final year at Cambridge, Madeleine (18) her first year at Warwick and Sam (13) was a pupil at the local comp. We had grandchildren too. My stepson Simon and his wife Maddy had two fantastic little girls; my stepdaughter Lucy and her husband Craig were just about to adopt a bouncing baby boy. Life was good.

On Christmas Day 2016, we were staying at my childhood home in the West Country with my parents and lots of family. Like many, our day revolved around a delicious meal, presents, jollity and merriment. We had absolutely no idea that a huge juggernaut of life-threatening illness was already hurtling towards us.

The star of this story is Alan, but for reasons that will become clear, he is not its narrator.

2017 was a year that changed our family forever, and nearly every day I found out something new. This is a book that gathers everything I learnt about coping with illness: the good, the bad, the funny, the sad and (I hope) the helpful.

Chapter One

BEGINNING

One moment in time

7PM BOXING DAY. A warm sitting room in Gloucestershire, filled with happiness, relatives and a certain degree of muddle. The debris of recently unwrapped presents, four or five dogs cantering around crazily, drinks being poured, a supper of roast ham and red cabbage (a family favourite) cooking. My husband stands, convivial as always, reading out loud an amusing letter from the newspaper. My daughters and I are laughing, it's funny, he's funny – we're all wrapped in a warm glow of familiarity and love. He gets to the last line – the punch line we think – and then his face, normally so animated, grimaces briefly and freezes. In that micro-second, I begin to say that this is in bad taste, not funny, why are you pretending to... I start to turn away crossly and, as I do, he falls, like a tree chopped down at the roots, his total collapse broken only partially by me. Within moments, his face turns dark blue. And at that exact moment, the earth tips and we all slide into a parallel universe.

Chaos

Eight months earlier, at the primary school where I worked as a learning support assistant, I did a first aid course. We role-played this exact situation: a person collapses (much hilarity when this part was enacted with some drama by a colleague), so what happens next? Now as Alan sprawls on the floor, utterly motionless, and my daughters start to scream, I feel as if I am back in that classroom with the St John Ambulance trainer standing next to me. I also feel as if I am looking at myself from somewhere very far away – watching someone who seems to know exactly what to do. 'Call an ambulance,' I tell my sister, Alice. 'Get everyone out the way, stand back, don't crowd him.' I roll my husband onto his back. He is incredibly heavy, a dead weight. Check for breathing, check for a pulse. There is none. His face is still a dark, purply blue. I can hear shouting and crying but it sounds as if it is underwater and, weirdly, I can also hear people laughing and chatting next door – not everyone has realised what is happening. I find the spot in the middle of his chest, put one hand on top of the other and start pressing down. One, two, three, four... I remember the instructions: two a second, press harder than you think, count to 30. Alan feels exactly like the training dummy – solid, rubbery, lifeless.

Then suddenly he gurgles – a deep shuddering roar as if he is a rock splitting in two. His face becomes pink, red, creased in some internal agony. He pushes up against my hands and then lurches down and immediately starts snoring. Thunderous snoring, frightening snoring – he seems possessed by some mighty force. I roll him onto his side, the recovery position. I shout at him, trying to wake him. By now, Alice has the ambulance service on the phone; she holds the receiver to my ear. Yes, he's breathing.

No, it isn't normal breathing. They advise me to start CPR again, but as soon as I try, he rises up with a growl: flailing, pushing, bellowing. 'Keep him lying down,' the ambulance lady says. 'We're on our way.' I can't hold him; my brother and brother-in-law have to restrain him. It is as if an angry bear has somehow blundered into the small sitting room. Then he crashes down again, motionless once more, his face clamped in pain, his mouth pressed shut. I try to open it – I can see that he is biting his tongue – and then he slumps and sags.

I have no idea how long this has been going on, but I hear someone shouting that they can see blue lights; the ambulance is here. Two paramedics stride in; they seem to have an enormous amount of medical paraphernalia and the house seems much too full of people, dogs and Christmas clutter to fit them in. They are authoritative, quite bossy in fact – reassuringly so. I want to find my three children – give them a hug and tell them Dad's going to be fine – but I daren't leave his side for a moment. But he looks better – he is sitting on the sofa now; he seems utterly bewildered and exhausted. 'We're taking him to hospital,' say the paramedics. 'You'll need to come in a car.'

Alice says that she'll drive me, and I'm trying to find my shoes, my coat, my handbag. People try and help but keep giving me the wrong things. My mum, a town councillor, is now chatting to the paramedics about the local air ambulance service. I want to tell her to stop holding them up – doesn't she realise this is an emergency? – but at the same time I am glad of the slight delay, as I am now panicking that if we don't leave exactly when the ambulance does, we'll lose them on the ten-mile drive into town. Later, my daughters tell me that the paramedics told them on the way out that 'Your dad's going to be alright, he's in good hands,' which meant a huge amount to them. Just before we leave, I dash around looking for my son, Sam. He is sitting in another room with his cousins, his head in his hands, sobbing. 'He's going to be OK,' I say. 'I know,' he says, rubbing his eyes. 'It's alright.' It isn't.

Driving

Alice pulls out directly behind the ambulance, and we follow it as it takes the twists and turns of the country lanes that lead to the larger main road and on towards the hospital. 'He's going to be alright,' my sister says. 'You were brilliant. You saved his life.' 'Don't lose the ambulance,' I say. 'I'm worried we'll get lost. Are you sure you know the way?' I think that Alan may have had a stroke, and I know that if he has, there is a high chance that he will have another one. 'They haven't got the blue lights on,' says Alice. 'That must be a good sign.' Just then, the ambulance puts the blue lights on. 'Oh god,' I say. We're on the A road now, and everyone local knows that the speed limit of 40mph is strictly enforced. 'Don't lose it,' I say. 'Just keep going.' A traffic light in front of us turns red; it's for a small side road to access the main road but we can see there are no cars on it. 'Keep going, keep going,' I say. Alice's face is set, she presses her lips together and runs the red light.

Nevertheless, the ambulance pulls further and further in front until we can't see the blue light anymore. As we get closer to the hospital, there are masses of roundabouts and all the road signs seem to jump in front of my eyes, but Alice is completely in control and pulls up in front of the main door. 'You run in. I'll park.' I skid across the floor and try and convey to the woman at the desk the urgency of the situation. I am panicking, thinking: what if he has had another attack? What if he has died on the way? What if I never see him alive again? What will I do without him? What if this is it, the end of us? She can't find his name on any list, and I start to think that maybe we've come to the wrong hospital. Then she realises that his details haven't actually been processed yet. Alice has driven so fast that we've arrived before the ambulance. 'He's just coming in now,' she says. 'Have a seat over there.'

I sit down as Alice runs in, and I explain what's happening. 'I'll just get you some water,' she says, and as she walks over to the water cooler, the oddest thing happens. I hear someone start to cry, properly cry, with ear-splitting, racking sobs, more like howling really. And I'm looking down from the ceiling, and I can see that the person down there sitting on a blue chair wailing loudly is me. And I can see my sister's head whip round, and then she's running back towards me, and the cup of water she's carrying is going absolutely everywhere. The receptionist has stood up and she's coming out from behind her desk; other people are staring. 'It's the shock,' says Alice, with her arm round me. 'It's just the shock. It's the shock.' 'He's OK,' says the receptionist. 'They're just bringing him in now, he's talking, he's OK.' Alice asks if we can just see him, and we go around the back of the desk to an ambulance bay where Alan is waiting on a bed. He smiles wanly as two burly men manoeuvre him into a small curtained area of a large room, full of bustle and drama.

The next couple of hours pass in a blur, with a series of procedures and tests. A doctor finally concludes that he has had some sort of seizure and tells us that it could well be a one-off: 'just one of those things'. He says that we can go home that night and just need to check in with our GP the following week. I take the first of what will be many (although I don't know it at the time) little videos on my phone of Alan, and WhatsApp it to the family. They tell me afterwards that they knew he was back to normal, because he says in the video that he has had a good trip in 'a Mercedes ambulance' – it is entirely typical of him to notice the make. Alice is talking on her phone to my mum, who asks to speak to me. She is worrying that we have missed supper and wants to tell me what there is to eat when we get back home. I am 53 years old. I am standing in the middle of a busy emergency ward and I have just saved my husband's life. I don't really think that now is the time for a lesson in how to heat up cabbage, but I listen to her, nonetheless.

Back to normal?

The first fallout from all the drama is the news that Alan will not be able to drive for at least a year. Alan minds this intensely and sits morosely in an armchair by the fireside at my parents' house, preoccupied with worry as to how he will cope. He has driven, and driven well, for over 50 years. His first job was in a car showroom in Croydon, then he drove lorries, then he became a sales rep in the north and, even when his job became more office based, driving to see customers was always one of the things he enjoyed most. His company car is the only perk that he values, he is a member of the Institute of Advanced Motorists and there probably haven't been many days since he was 17 when he hasn't been behind the wheel. Almost all our holidays have included him driving a car. He has driven me up the west coast of America in a convertible; he has driven to Berlin to move his eldest son Simon into a flat; he has driven Sam and a carload of 11-year-old mates to France for a football tournament; the summer before, he drove the five of us on a family road trip across France, Belgium,

Germany, Switzerland and Italy. And he has loved every single minute. He never drove again after that first seizure in 2016, but still, to this very day, he believes himself to be a driver, often thinking that he has just come back from a trip. We have come to realise that it is as if driving is so deeply wired into his DNA that his brain can't unlearn it.

The day after the first seizure, while Alan has been plunged into gloom about not driving, I am already learning three lessons that will come to characterise the next 12 months. First, I am going to have to step up. Alan's company car in which he has transported us to Gloucestershire is a fairly new, large, seven-seater estate. I drive a little 20-year-old Nissan Micra with no power steering and have never driven anything big or modern. Most of my driving is short journeys related to picking up kids and, in fact, there are lots of days when I don't drive at all, which is fine by me as I don't especially like driving! Now, I am going to have to get this monster of a company car back up the wintery motorway, and the prospect completely terrifies me. My immediate thought is quite simply that I can't do it. One of Alan's sales team will have to get themselves down here and drive us back home. Then I have a firm word with myself. If I have saved someone's life, surely driving a large car along a motorway must be within my capabilities.

Second, I am going to need bottomless reserves of optimism. I tell Alan that it's fine: I'm going to be able to drive him to work, his reps can drive him to see his customers, he can get taxis, we live in a city where there is plenty of public transport. However, a little voice inside me is saying that this is going to be a total nightmare. Alan has never been a very good passenger, and if I'm spending my time driving him around, how am I ever going to have a career of my own again? Is my life about to become that of an unpaid chauffeur? I squash the little voice down, deep inside my tummy, underneath my fears about driving his car, and carry on telling Alan that everything will be OK.

And third, it is fortunate that we don't know what the future holds for us. If I had realised on that day how very much worse things were going to get, I would never have had the strength for the first two lessons.

Home

The drive back is in thick fog and, thanks to terrible traffic, it is dark by the time we're home. Due to the unfamiliar gearbox, I've stalled several times before we're even ten metres from my parents' house. Alan is tense, I'm exhausted and the kids are scratchy. But we're home in one piece, and the car is unscathed. I park it outside our front door and breathe. Over the next few days, life trundles on. We are in that odd limbo between Christmas and new year, when real life stops and you eat meals largely composed of cold meat, brandy butter, bread sauce and small jars of chutney.

We check in with our GP. Although Dr Marber is chatty and reassuring, jolly even, I experience the same sinking sensation that I felt when talking to the doctors at the hospital. Speaking on behalf of another adult feels weird and wrong. Alan now seems perfectly well, but he can't remember anything at all about his collapse, so I have to talk for him, and it feels unpleasantly like taking one of our children to the doctor. Already the balance of our partnership is tipping, although I have no idea how far the scales have yet to fall. Dr Marber checks Alan's blood pressure, asks a few questions and says that he seems completely fine. A one-off collapse is not unusual – perhaps Alan has been working too hard – and we agree that, yes, the run-up to the Christmas break is always very busy. The medical consensus seems to be that one seizure doesn't mean anything sinister. As we leave, Alan asks if there is anything he should do. 'Just make sure you don't have another one...ha ha ha,' says Dr Marber.

Happy Hogmanay

A few days later, it's New Year's Eve and, unusually, all of us have parties to go to. Alan, Sam and I are all invited to dinner with our good pals Annie and Andy. They are brilliant hosts, the house is nearby so we can walk, we've bought a big box of fireworks, there will be a small group of teenagers Sam's age together with their parents who we all know well and it should be lots of fun. The girls are both off to different parties with friends. They look super-glamorous, and I hustle them into the sitting room with Sam to pose for some photos next to the Christmas tree. We're larking about and then one of us says, 'Come on, family selfie, let's get Dad in here too.' We shout for him and then suddenly look at each other. 'Where actually is Dad?' I say I think he's next door in the study, and then Madeleine, who has dashed through, shouts out in alarm. It's happened again; this time he's clearly fallen off a chair, which has tipped over. It's hard to get to him as the room is cramped, and he must have hit his head on the cast-iron mantelpiece as he fell, so there's blood. He's semi-conscious, moaning and not really able to speak, and he doesn't seem to understand what's happening. The ambulance comes quickly, and this time I can go in it with him. To my surprise, once we're inside, the ambulance stays parked for a while, and the crew ask me which hospital I want him to go to. This is the first of many occasions when medical professionals will present me with decisions that I feel entirely unqualified to make. In this instance, I blurt out that surely we should go to the closest one, but the crew explain that since the ambulance is itself a pretty sophisticated mini-hospital, they have everything they need to keep Alan alive and I have time to consider. I still choose the nearest one and, with a huge dollop of hindsight, this is in fact a mistake. The hospital he starts off in doesn't have a neurology department, and waiting for a bed and a transfer to the larger hospital some weeks later takes an agonising length of time. But on that cold, dark December evening, I couldn't have possibly known this, and at the time, speed seemed to be the most important thing.

Within ten minutes we are there and I am standing with Alan, who is now conscious, as he waits on a trolley in a cramped and chaotic corridor for a bed in the emergency ward. On the trolley next to him is an elderly Irishman, plainly the worse for drink, complaining loudly about how much pain his legs are in and how long things are taking. The staff obviously know him; they remonstrate with him almost affectionately, roll their eyes and carry on trying to find space for patients on what is going to be a very busy night. The Irishman moves on to his own history: he has spent most of his life in the army, he laments the lack of support, the absence of respect, the loss of dignity. Alan sits up, reaches over and clasps the man's hand. 'You're a hero. A hero,' he says. 'Don't forget.' The man's eyes fill with tears, and I am overwhelmed with admiration for my husband's ability to empathise with someone else, even when his own circumstances are far from good. This is one of the first things I learn in hospital: there will always be someone worse off than you, and helping them will help you.

Midnight, 31 December 2016

The staff find a bed for Alan, in a cubicle right in the middle of the emergency ward, where we have an excellent view of what a highly demanding night's work looks like in a large city hospital. It's strangely absorbing, like being on the set of *ER* or *Casualty*, and the feeling that we have somehow wandered onto a TV location contributes to my general sense of unreality. As before, Alan now appears to be back to normal following the seizure, but he can't remember what's happened. With hindsight, I can see that his brain wasn't really processing what was going on, but at the time he just seemed extremely tired. The doctors are running blood tests and doing CT scans, and it's all going to take time. I am so grateful that Alan is in a bed and surrounded by reassuring machines and nurses that I don't actually care how long it takes, and spending New Year's Eve here almost seems quite fun – a bit of an adventure.

I phone the kids, who are back at home, anxiously waiting for news, and let them know that although Dad now seems OK, we are likely to be here for a while. I persuade the girls that they may as well go out with their friends, and Al's sister Ginny and her husband Tim look after Sam. They order an Indian takeaway and watch a *Harry Potter* film.

Meanwhile, the emergency ward is getting fuller and fuller. Just before midnight, a jolly nurse comes around with some plastic cups and a bottle of non-alcoholic champagne. I take a selfie of the two of us 'clinking' our cups, with the emergency ward clock in the background, the hands at exactly midnight. As the 'Happy New Year' messages and social media posts start to flood in to my phone, I feel a disconcerting disconnect between what seem to be two entirely separate worlds. Is the real world the one that is going on out there, with fireworks, fun and festivity? Or is the real world here, in the curtained cubicle with my sleeping husband and a gently bleeping machine?

As yet, I have no idea that Izzy, Madeleine, Sam and I are going to spend the whole of 2017 occupying this strange twilight zone – constantly travelling through portals between one universe and another. The next morning, the doctors discharge Alan, with a probable diagnosis of epilepsy, some super-strong anti-seizure pills and an appointment at a clinic in a few weeks' time.

January 2017

The new year begins with an odd mix of normal and not-quite-normal. Sam goes back to school and Madeleine goes back to uni. I drive her to Warwick in Alan's big car so that we can take all her stuff, and I feel surprisingly confident – the car is easier to manoeuvre than I anticipated, although I still keep on stalling it. Izzy's Cambridge term starts in a fortnight, and I feel confident that this drive too will be within my capabilities. Alan goes back to work. I drive him there and back, and we agree that this is all completely do-able. It takes me about 20 minutes each way; this is not going to be a problem.

There's a new job for me, too. Since the previous autumn, I have been launching a fledgling career as a copywriter, writing websites and brochures for various small businesses. A meeting with a potential new client this week goes well, and I am energised; there's lots of work to do and the pay is good. There's a tiny amount of snow and as usual everyone, including me, gets overly excited.

But at the same time, small nagging things are happening

that are not quite so positive. One evening, sitting in the kitchen, Alan says, 'It's funny, but I feel as if I've never been here before.' Another time, he suggests we go outside to the swimming pool. We look out at our small, frosty, paved garden and then back at him, confused. We watch *Blade Runner*, one of his favourite films, and he doesn't seem to follow the plot at all, even though he's seen it many times. I ask him to change a light bulb, and he stands there staring at the fitting, unable to work out quite what he needs to do, and then storms off crossly when I impatiently ask him what on earth's going on. We have an arrangement that at 5:45pm every evening, when I pick him up from his office, he will wait for me by the fire escape door in the car park. But every day he waits somewhere different; one day he's actually walking down the middle of the road and leaps into my car as if it is a total coincidence that I was driving past. His voice is changing too: it's oddly slurry, almost sluggish. It's hard to put my finger on, but he's definitely not quite himself. (Much later, his two colleagues in the office, Pat and Nuala, will tell me that during those ten days, they were increasingly concerned about his erratic behaviour. And then, a great deal later, I will see the emails that he has sent to customers and clients during that first fortnight in January and be shocked to realise how rambling and nonsensical they were.)

Entirely understandably, Al says he's finding it very hard to come to terms with the concept of having epilepsy, and I channel my feelings of apprehension into showing him helpful websites and sending off for endless booklets and leaflets. Bizarrely, he can't seem to remember the actual word 'epilepsy'. He keeps writing it down on Post-it notes, which I find in his pockets, and his writing, though never particularly legible at the best of times, has now become tiny. Epilepsy. The little word looks like a spell or a charm, it's all a bit strange. Maybe the strong tablets he's taking are making him a bit weird? I take the folded bit of paper listing the possible side effects from the packet of his medication and uneasily scan the small print. The list is very long and hard to make much sense of. Drowsiness is mentioned, as are irritability and clumsiness. Maybe that's it. And I can ask the doctor at the epilepsy clinic that Alan's booked in to attend in a few weeks' time. So, we try to get on with our lives and move forward, despite an underlying feeling of slight disquiet. No one says – stop, something's not quite right here, what's going on?

Third time unlucky

We might not be saying 'stop', but the malevolent forces at work inside Alan's brain certainly are. On Friday the 13th of January I get a call from Nuala in the office to say it's happened again, and Al is being rushed into hospital. Just as before, there has been no warning: one minute he's working on his computer, the next he's unconscious on the floor. The staff in the large serviced office where he works have been fantastic, first aiders were summoned, an ambulance was called.

I meet Alan back in the same emergency ward that we were in on New Year's Eve. This time, things are not quite so jolly. Alan doesn't seem quite so recovered as he did before, and my faith in the system is starting to wobble a bit. Why, if he is on anti-seizure medication, is he still having seizures? How likely is it that a 66-year-old man with no previous health issues would suddenly develop epilepsy? Why am I answering exactly the same questions every time we arrive in hospital – surely his records must be on a computer somewhere? Is it possible that no one here actually knows what's wrong with him?

He stays in for another night, and the next morning I come back to see what the doctors have to say on their morning rounds. When they hear about his forthcoming appointment at the epilepsy clinic, they are clearly relieved. Phew, we can move on. The system is working fine, this patient now seems perfectly OK to go home and, anyway, he's booked in for another appointment, so he won't feel that we've given up on him completely. Hurrah, someone else will soon be dealing with this slightly strange set of symptoms and his annoyingly persistent wife.

Then, as we wait to be discharged, a tall doctor with a clever and kind but furrowed face hangs back to talk to me. 'There's something not quite right here,' he says. I feel a lurch of dread-relief, an emotion that soon becomes all too familiar – a peculiar mix of 'oh no' and 'thank goodness'. These are not the words that anyone wants to hear, but how glad I am that someone medical is vocalising what I sense. 'I'm booking him in to the TIA clinic on Monday,' he continues. TIA? I don't know what it stands for, but I do know that it means a stroke and the terror surges up. That had been my first thought back on Boxing Day and is the thing that frightens me the most. I stammer that surely a stroke has been ruled out – they've done scans, run tests. He looks at me steadily. 'It's not a stroke,' he says. 'But he needs to be seen by someone.' Afterwards, I realise that what he's really saying is 'by someone who knows more about brains', and this hospital doesn't have a neurology department. Weeks later, I bump into the same doctor in the hospital café and am happy to be there to see the look of pleasure spread across his tired face when I confirm that his instincts were bang on – something was indeed 'not quite right'.

Monday morning at the TIA (transient ischemic attack) clinic

We arrive in good time for our 10am appointment. I am armed with a list of things to ask that I've been writing down all weekend, and I feel that now, finally, we will get to the bottom of this. I anticipate seeing a bespectacled, brainy-looking doctor in a small calm office, who will immediately diagnose Alan with something unusual but solvable. We won't be having noisy conversations with harassed junior doctors who perch on the end of beds, we won't be surrounded by busy nurses taking endless blood samples. I have sensible questions and there will be sensible answers; this will be dealt with by experts.

To my extreme annoyance, I find that even after quite a lengthy wait, we are not allowed to see the actual doctor until we have been 'triaged' by a large bossy woman, to whom I take an instant dislike. I explain pleasantly that we do have an appointment and that she does already have all of Alan's details on file. But there is no getting past her, and something about her questions implies that she thinks Alan is here under false pretences and that he's going to be wasting her boss's time. Everything she asks Alan – his name, date of birth and so on – he answers correctly, and I can see her thinking that this does not look like someone who has anything whatsoever wrong with them. And he palpably hasn't had a stroke.

Then she asks Alan why he's here and, without missing a beat, Alan says, 'Well, we're all here for the Sales Conference of course.' It's almost comical. Her jaw literally drops, and she says, 'Pardon me? Where are we?' 'At the conference hotel,' Alan says patiently, as if she's the one with the problem. 'In Edinburgh,' he adds helpfully. She looks at me, and I stare right back. Inside I am panicking, thinking, 'What? WHAT? He thinks he's in Edinburgh?' But I'm also triumphant. 'See. SEE. Something's not right here. Now DO something about it.' After that, things happen very fast. We see the doctor, and she asks a lot more questions, many of which Alan answers with utterly nonsensical responses. This time, he says we're in Bristol, in an airport lounge. She doesn't know what's causing this confusion, although she's certain it's not a stroke, but she decides that she will admit him 'for a few days' so that they can try and find out. I was not expecting this and embark on a flurry of texts and phone calls to get Sam to pack an overnight bag for his dad and Annie to bring it to us.

At this point, my understanding of the workings of the NHS are sadly optimistic. When the doctor says she's going to admit him, I envisage us walking down a flight of stairs and straight onto a ward. Instead, she tells us it is the current policy to check in patients via the A&E department. This is right down in the bowels of the building, and when we get there, it is total chaos. We are told that it could be an eight-hour wait for a bed, during which time we will be sitting in a very narrow, very busy corridor. In fact, we are lucky to have chairs. Alan finally gets a bed at 8pm. It is the 16th of January, and the 'few days' that I think Alan might be in hospital for will stretch into an eternity. He will not come home again until the 29th of November.

Waiting

I arrive on the ward the next morning with an optimistic attitude. As before, I anticipate that soon I will see a specialist doctor, who will answer all my questions. However, I have not factored in two major issues. First, before anyone even starts to diagnose what's wrong, there will be a multitude of tests and scans. And one scan, the MRI of his brain, will not be happening any time soon, as this is a scanner that has a department, a team of operators and a waiting list all of its own. Getting the MRI scan soon acquires an almost mythical status for us; it seems that if we can just see inside Alan's brain, it will be obvious what's wrong. We wait for almost a week, but when he finally has the scan it is disappointingly inconclusive.

Meanwhile, as well as the many other tests and scans, there are endless questions, many of which Alan cannot sensibly answer. Almost imperceptibly, I have become his spokesperson. Again and again, they ask me about previous illnesses, excessive drinking and recreational drug use. To me, these questions are all very odd, especially since the answer to all of them is a resounding, 'No, no, none.' It almost feels to me that they don't believe my answers, which I find stressful and infuriating.

Months later, when I understand much more about how doctors function, I see that of course they are looking for the most likely solution to the symptoms they are presented with, not the most improbable. And the possible causes for the confusion and incoherence they are witnessing in this 66-year-old man could be alcoholism, drug use or epilepsy. It is much less likely to be an uncommon ailment.

So, the days go by and they carry on testing and questioning, until they reach a conclusion. And that brings us to the second issue – that this hospital doesn't have a neurology department – so seeing an expert becomes a new challenge. They tell us that a consultant has been booked to come and talk to us.

———

Chapter Two

A DIAGNOSIS

The answer?

W E WAIT. DAYS GO by. I drive in every morning and sit by Alan's bed all day, chatting to him, the nurses and the other patients, while waiting to see the legendary expert on whom we are now pinning all our hopes. Alan is strangely calm. We are all so worried and focused on the next step that we don't entirely notice that he is not really engaging normally with the world around him or stop to wonder why he's sleeping so much.

Finally, the fabled neurologist arrives. He is balding, bespectacled and brainy, and reminds the kids and me of the evil Swedish mastermind in a recent episode of *Sherlock*. He asks Alan many questions, and this time they are questions designed to find out what is going on in his brain, not enquiries about his lifestyle. I am horrified to see that he cannot count back from 100. He cannot remember a sentence for two minutes. He cannot think of five words beginning with 'a' – in fact, he cannot think of one. He has no idea where he is. Dr Super Smart tells me that he's pretty sure that what Alan has is encephalitis. I have never heard this word before but I discover it means inflammation or swelling of the brain, from the Greek word 'encephalo' meaning brain and 'itis' meaning inflammation. There are three main causes of encephalitis: a viral infection, a bacterial infection or an autoimmune reaction. The first two are relatively easy to treat; the autoimmune type is not so simple. He hopes that some strong antiviral medication or antibiotics will do the trick. Finally, we have a diagnosis and a plan, and everyone feels a lot more positive. But then Alan has another seizure.

Through the fog

It is 8:15am and I'm having breakfast in the kitchen with Sam before he goes to school. He's just about to leave, and we're chatting away about my plan for the day and hoping that Alan might be quite a bit better when I go into the ward later that morning.

Just as he is about to walk out the door, the phone rings. It's the hospital. A nurse tells me that Alan has just had a seizure and this time he's not regaining consciousness. She thinks I should come in immediately. I can't properly process what she's telling me; a white noise seems to fill my head and I'm struggling to hear her. 'But, but – my son's here with me. Are you saying...? What are you saying...? Do you mean...? Do you think I should bring him too?' An infinitesimal pause. She sounds as if she's looking at someone else for confirmation. 'Yes. Yes, I think you should. You need to get here as soon as you can.' Sam can see from my face that it's bad news. I don't want him to know that his dad might be dying, might already be dead, but I know I can't easily reassure him, can't tell him something that isn't true. In fact, there's absolutely nothing I can say to him apart from what the nurse has just told me.

We run out to my car and drive immediately into the morning traffic jam on the flyover. There is thick fog and it is still quite dark. It is also absolutely freezing and, to make matters worse, a couple of days earlier, the driver's window of my ancient little car jammed open, so our icy breath mingles with exhaust fumes. We crawl along, watching the red lights stretching out ahead of us. We are silent. We both know there is nothing we can say that will make the other person feel any better, and there is nothing we can do to go any faster.

When we get to the hospital, we run through the foyer and up the stairs. I am incredibly worried about what we will find, about what Sam might see, but I can't think of anything else apart from getting to Alan as quickly as possible. We sprint onto the ward, and he's there, in a different bed, but he's awake, he recognises us, he's talking. He is much less aware than he was yesterday, but the relief of not finding him dead is indescribable. There is an air of calm after a storm – doctors are moving around quietly, monitors are bleeping gently. A nurse explains that they are concerned that the seizures seem to be getting more frequent and severe. The plan is now to transfer him to a much larger hospital that has a dedicated neurology ward just as soon as a bed becomes available. For the first time since this began, I properly begin to appreciate that this could be a much longer process than I could have ever imagined.

A different neurology consultant gives me the unwelcome news that since Alan is not getting any better, they are starting to think that the encephalitis is caused by his own immune system malfunctioning and not by an infection. This means that it will be much more complicated to treat. 'But you can treat it?' I ask. Her mouth tightens. 'It is difficult,' she says. 'It will take time.' 'How much time?' I ask. She looks at me. I know by now that doctors don't like guessing. 'Well, give me some idea,' I plead. 'Are we talking days, weeks, months...years?' 'Months,' she says, 'many months.' I stare at her, aghast.

Nil by mouth

Another morning. I sit by Alan's bed, and the day drags slowly on. A nurse tells me that they have put in a catheter. I only really know what a catheter is because I had one following my caesarean to have Izzy, and that was because I wasn't allowed to get out of bed. Why does Alan have one? Can't he walk? No one seems to be sure. No one seems to be saying what is only obvious to me with hindsight: that his ability to do normal things is rapidly slipping away. And because no one is really saying it, it feels as if it isn't actually happening.

Alan is sleeping most of the time; when he wakes up, he smiles at me and says, 'Hi babe,' but his voice is thick and dopey. I assume it is the medication. As well as the catheter, he has a thin tube taped into a vein in his hand and a rubber thimble on his finger, which seems to be measuring his heart rate. Both of these he constantly tries to take off, picking and pulling as if they are leeches. 'No, leave them on Alan,' say the nurses; he smiles vaguely and then starts tugging at them again. It's annoying and also frightening: why is he behaving so weirdly? Another nurse arrives with what looks like yogurt. She tries to spoon it into his mouth, but it's going everywhere; he can't seem to swallow or move his tongue out of the way of the spoon.

Suddenly, a doctor sweeps in on her morning rounds, with a small cohort of acolytes scurrying behind her to push the laptop trolley and draw the curtains round the bed. She takes one look and says officiously, 'Nil by mouth. This patient should be nil by mouth. Write it on the board please.' I gasp in horror and then burst into loud tears. Nil by mouth is a terrifying phrase that I associate with TV dramas and paraplegics. How dare she use it so casually. She frowns at me. 'Can someone take this lady to another room please, she's clearly very upset and she shouldn't be here.' I recover fast. I'm not going anywhere. 'I'm upset,' I say loudly and deliberately, 'because that is a totally unacceptable way to talk to a patient.' The other medical staff look at each other; the doctor looks flustered and then suggests we go into another room. 'You can talk to me here,' I say. 'I'm his wife.' She consults notes, talks to colleagues, gives me the usual medical flimflam that I have heard for the last few days: 'We're running more tests, assessing, these things are complicated, they all take time.' Then in a lower voice she says to the ward nurse, 'Get the ICU assessment team up here right now.' That night, Alan is moved to the intensive-care unit (ICU), and a day later, he is in a coma.

Chapter Three

A MATTER OF LIFE AND DEATH

The brink

THE ICU IS AN intense mix of extreme tranquillity and high drama. There is no natural light at all, and it feels very far from normality. The beds are much further apart than on the general ward, and each one has a dizzying array of technology surrounding it. Every patient has their own individual nurse, and seated at the foot of each bed, calm and kind, they seem to me to be literal guardian angels, watching over their charges. You can sense immediately that life hangs in the balance here. During the week that Alan is in the ICU, when the beds around him become empty, we know that it is not always because people have got better.

Alan is connected to almost every machine you can imagine. There is a tube running to a ventilator to keep him breathing, there is a feeding tube down his nose, there are endless fluid lines and wires running from his body to drip stands and monitors that bleep and flash. They are reassuring but also alarming; everyone has seen too many medical dramas not to jump whenever the bleeping speeds up or, even worse, stops. I look at the zigzag green and orange lines and hummocks on the screen and imagine them flattened, imagine the consistent bleeping becoming a drawn-out monotone. Alan lies motionless. The staff have given him a shave, and his normally bearded face looks defenceless and vulnerable. The scene reminds me of the chapter in *The Lion, the Witch and the Wardrobe*, in which Lucy and Susan find Aslan laid out on the stone table. The White Witch's minions have shaved off his fur and they think he is dead. My lion of a husband has been brought down by an invisible foe.

Only two visitors are allowed in at any one time, but the unit has its own waiting room in which families gather, each caught up in their own private dramas, but also talking quietly to each other, and there is a sense of camaraderie, of bonding – we are all in this together. Izzy and Madeleine have come home from university and Alan's two older children, Lucy and Simon, are here now too. Together with Sam, Ginny and Tim, we all come and go – in and out of the small waiting room, in and out of the ward. Normal life is suspended; we take it in turns to buy sandwiches, get coffees, cook supper, drive home and back, tell each other which buses to get, who's going to be at home and who has a key, cancel activities, relay information. It feels as if we are all part of the same person, all focused on the same purpose.

When I am sitting next to Alan, I talk and talk, prattling away about anything and everything. The nurse tells me she has never seen anyone talk so constantly to someone in a coma; she says it's a good thing. I feel a rush of emotion that I can still do something helpful when I am feeling so utterly helpless. The kids do the same, telling Alan about school, university, life. Sometimes I use my phone to play music to him, putting one headphone in his ear and one in mine, so we can listen to the same thing. As Bob

Dylan sings 'It ain't no use in callin' out my name, gal; I can't hear you anymore', I don't realise that I'm crying until the nurse passes me a tissue.

Days pass.

The doctors say that they think he could wake up, and we are instructed to talk loudly, almost bossily, commanding, 'Wake up Alan!' Again, I feel happy to be useful; loud and bossy is something I can definitely do. Simon records his two little girls, our granddaughters Nancy and Esther, who are five and nearly two, shouting 'Wake up Grandpa!' on his phone. They rise to the challenge superbly, and it is so deafening that we have to play it to Alan through headphones, so as not to disturb the other patients. For a few days there is no perceptible change. Then, the improvement is very gradual: his eyes start to flicker and occasionally open. And then, one morning, he's properly focusing; he looks bewildered but he's definitely present. I talk to him and, yes, he seems to know who I am and what I'm saying. I wish so much that the others were here to see him, and then I think to rummage in my bag for my phone and record him. I tell him how happy we are that he's back with us and ask if he could manage to move his hand and do a thumbs up. For a moment, it seems as if this is beyond him, his arm shakes and he looks confused, but then, slowly but surely, he puts his thumb up! Suddenly, a nurse comes over and nicely but firmly tells me that cameras are *not* allowed in the ICU. But I don't care, I've got my video. And when I send it to the family a few moments later, tearful messages of joy come flooding back.

The move

Once Alan is able to leave intensive care, the move to the specialist neurology ward at a larger hospital becomes imminent. I can tell from the way the doctors talk to me that there is a new sense of urgency, a feeling that he needs to be seen by experts as soon as possible. He's breathing, he's eating and he's talking, but his poor brain is utterly scrambled – he can't think of the words for everyday things, can't feed himself. And there's something else, something grim. Every half an hour or so his head turns slowly, as if he's looking over his left shoulder at someone who isn't there. Then his left hand starts twitching, scrabbling, picking at his hospital gown, increasingly frantically. He's aware he's doing it, but unable to stop, he says, 'I'm just...' or, 'I need to...' or, 'Where's...?' His entire body shudders as if possessed by some malignant force; it lasts for about ten minutes and then it stops. It's horrible and frightening. The doctors observe it but can offer no real explanation; it seems that they know they are out of their depth.

Later, the neurologists tell us that it is another type of seizure, and years afterwards, on a BBC drama, I see a man having an epileptic fit that starts with the same odd uncontrollable head turn to the left, the same inability to explain what's happening. But at the time, we know nothing of this, and it feels to us, as we watch this scary and ever-more-frequent phenomenon, that Alan has been taken over by something strange and sinister. He is moved to the high dependency unit, and the staff are wonderful, but it feels rather as if he is in a holding pattern, waiting for some insight, an expert, the cure. Finally, a nurse calls me at home one evening to say that, at last, he will be moving, and overnight he is transferred to the specialist neurology ward of a much larger hospital.

Chapter Four

A WHOLE
NEW WORLD

Bad luck, good luck

U NTIL ALAN FELL ILL, I had spent little time in hospital. Having three children and visiting elderly relatives were virtually my only experiences. But from January until May of 2017, I visited every day, sometimes twice a day. From June until November, when Alan was hospitalised on the other side of the city in a Brain Rehab Centre, I went in most days. By the end of the year, I had spent a significant part of it inside a hospital and Alan had spent 318 nights sleeping in a hospital bed.

We had joined an entire community whose members are linked mainly by a desire not to be there in the first place. And very few of us are even remotely prepared for it. The stats reveal that, in 2018–19, every day an average of 67,991 people attended A&E departments and over 13,000 people were admitted to hospital via A&E. Every day! In England, the NHS treats over a million of us every 36 hours. The numbers are truly staggering. The great paradox of hospitals is that we count ourselves unlucky to be inside one and yet in fact we are extraordinarily lucky. According to the World Health Organization, at least half of the world's population cannot obtain essential health services.

Someone like you

I've realised that if there is one thing that everyone has in common when they first go into a hospital, it is the feeling that 'this can't be happening to me'. That surreal, almost out-of-body experience is described time and time again, whether it's by a mother who goes into labour early, victims in an accident or a family like us for whom an unexpected doctor's diagnosis has led to a surreally swift pathway to a hospital ward.

What both patient and carer are experiencing is emotional shock. After a trauma, there is a lot that your mind needs to process before it can function properly, and with a sudden admission to hospital this time is often condensed, so that neither the relative nor the patient has time to adapt before the next bit of bad news. I would have found it helpful to acknowledge that my sense that it was all a horrible nightmare was completely normal.

For the first month or so, I still woke up every morning believing that the previous day's events had been a dream. Meanwhile, in my actual dreams, Alan was still fit and well. If you are talking to someone who has unexpectedly gone into hospital, I think it is useful to know that this feeling of disbelief and disorientation comes from genuine trauma and shouldn't be ignored. Do say 'This must be incredibly difficult, and I expect it hasn't properly sunk in yet.' Encourage them to talk about how they are feeling. Do not say 'I, oh, just know it will all work out, you have always been such a lucky and positive family.' Several friends said this to me almost immediately when Alan was taken into hospital, and I wanted to punch them. And I later discovered that this anger is also a symptom of shock.

Coping with trauma

If you or someone you love is suddenly taken ill, the emotional shock can cause post-traumatic stress. However horrendous that sounds, it is your body's normal reaction to an abnormal event, and knowing that can make it easier to deal with. Some of the things you may feel are:

- disbelief
- numbness
- fear
- vulnerability
- sadness
- anger

Some things that may well help are:

- talking
- rest
- routine
- time

How long has this been going on?

Back in the first hospital, on a general ward, while Alan is taken off for a scan, I start chatting to the woman who is visiting her husband in the bed opposite. In fact, before we meet, I hear her talking to him, behind the blue curtains that draw around each bed to give each patient privacy. They may shield the bed from view, but they do nothing to block out the sound and the rest of the ward, and I can clearly hear every word. She's trying to help him to use the commode to go to the toilet. He's obviously quite large as she's struggling to move him, and he's being extremely grumpy. She's very patient but she sounds utterly exhausted. The ward is pleasant enough, clean and warm, but I think how grim it is to have to do things like that in such a public place and resolve to get Alan back home as soon as possible.

When she draws back the curtain, I smile at her and she immediately starts talking. As I surmised, she is indeed thoroughly fed up, but I am surprised to hear that she doesn't want her husband to come home. She doesn't think she will be able to cope. I naively can't really contemplate how being on this ward can possibly be better than being in your own house and ask how long her husband has been here. When she tells me that tomorrow it will be 16 weeks, I almost fall off my chair. Sixteen weeks?! I work out that he must have come in way before Christmas, back in the autumn. I can't get my head around it.

We talk for ages, and I find out that her husband has been in a motorbike accident. She comes in to visit him every day, and although he is much improved, he is by no means fully recovered. But the hospital has now done all it can, so he has to go home. Is that how it works? If this grouchy man was my husband, I'm not sure I'd want him home either. I feel desperately sorry for her and tell her that I think she's doing a brilliant job. 'Thanks,' she says. 'Pity some people don't think so.'

Then I chat to the man in the bed next to Alan's. He is elderly but seems fit; he's clever and sprightly. So, why's he here? I find out he has sprained his wrist. Is that all? Now I feel sorry for myself, not this man who knows nothing of trauma, of seizures. He's an imposter. But then he goes on to say that the reason he's here is that he lives alone and can't manage with one arm. And the reason he lives alone is that his wife died last month. Of leukaemia. 'Oh yes, I know this hospital well,' he says sadly. 'I was in every day for months. I just didn't think I'd be back again so soon.'

Both the grumpy man and the sprightly man have gone the next morning and of course I never see them again. But I am left with an awareness of three things. First, you cannot make assumptions about other people's illnesses. Second, the concept of time in hospital is very different to that in the outside world. And third, a lot of people's lives are much tougher than yours.

The rhythm of life

Once Alan has his bed on the neurology ward, I settle into a kind of routine. It seems extraordinary to think of it like that, when every day is stressful and no two days are the same, yet having a kind of pattern to the days makes me feel calmer and more purposeful. The girls are back at university, Sam is at school and of course they visit as much as they can, as do other relations. I always go in in the mornings, to try and be there when the doctors do their rounds. To start with, I stay by Alan's bedside all day, but as the weeks stretch into months, I see that this is not sustainable.

And in the early days, I am desperate for progress, action, results, but gradually, I become accustomed to the pace of 'hospital time'. I discover that the neurology team have meetings every Friday, and this is where the big decisions are made. I discover that absolutely nothing happens at weekends, and the building is so deserted during the April and May bank holidays that it is as if some sort of apocalypse has occurred. I discover that the doctors are on a rota, so the doctor you see on Monday will never be the one you see on Tuesday. Some doctors I have lengthy conversations with and then never see again. But the nurses, cleaners, porters and other staff on the ward become like friends. Every day, the same ward receptionist says good morning, the same lovely nurse wheels the medications trolley down the corridor and tells me what sort of night Alan has had, the same smiley girl takes the order for Alan's food, the same chatty cleaner mops his floor and the same friendly housekeeper changes his bedsheets and water jugs. And they all know him, talk to him, help him. I marvel at the sheer number of people who have become an integral part of Alan's care.

Perhaps most important of all are the RMNs – the registered nurses trained in mental health – who are assigned to look after him. He quickly becomes too disruptive for a ward and is moved to his own room and then also given one-to-one care, both for his own safety and that of the other patients. These nurses sit with him in his small room all day and all night. They are patient, they are kind, they are professional. But sometimes Alan doesn't like them. It soon becomes apparent that if he takes a dislike to a nurse, things do not go well. He becomes rude and angry, incidents occur, official forms are filled in and I worry that they will insist that he leaves. On other days, I arrive to find him affable and relaxed, chatting to an RMN who exudes chilled laid-back vibes and, inevitably, Alan's mood becomes calmer and happier too. Every day is different and yet also the same.

Assume nothing

It takes me a long time to discover how doctors actually find out what's wrong with you. Before Alan was ill, I think I assumed that the process went something like this. A doctor studies for seven years to learn as much medicine as they can. A patient arrives with symptoms. The doctor makes a good guess, based on their own knowledge and what they can find out from examining and talking to the patient. Tests then confirm this diagnosis, and the doctor proceeds to treat the patient accordingly. Sometimes, I imagined (as in TV dramas), the doctor makes a truly inspired deduction based on coincidental information that they have miraculously accumulated.

In fact, the actual process is much more mundane than this and also much slower. But, as I gradually come to appreciate, it has a much better chance of being accurate. First, a good doctor will assume absolutely nothing. There's a phrase (which I think originated in an old American TV sitcom, *The Odd Couple*), 'Never assume, because when you assume, you make an ASS of U and ME', and this appears to be the motto of doctors too. In the beginning, I found it frustrating that the doctors didn't seem to believe me when I said that of course Alan wasn't an alcoholic, of course he hadn't taken large quantities of hallucinogenic drugs and of course something like this had never happened before; but I see now that they couldn't assume that.

Second, doctors do not want to tell you what they are thinking while they are working it out. This, again, is incredibly frustrating. We kept saying 'But what do you think is wrong with him?' and 'What could be causing these symptoms?' and no one would say anything other than 'It's too early to know.' But if a doctor decides too soon what the illness might be, there is a danger that they will make their own diagnosis fit in with this theory and miss something else. A doctor doesn't jump to a conclusion, they move towards it using very small, measured steps.

Third, instead of wondering what it *could* be, doctors proceed very methodically to rule out what it *couldn't* be. In Alan's case, blood tests told them he wasn't having a heart attack, a CT scan told them he hadn't had a stroke and an MRI scan told them he didn't have a brain tumour. They could see he was having seizures, and they could also see he was extremely confused. Encephalitis is not common, and in fact, one doctor blithely said to me that 50 years ago the diagnosis would have probably been 'unexplained madness'.

Once they reached a possible diagnosis, it then, again, seemed to be an agonisingly slow process to find out what sort of encephalitis he had. First, a blood test ruled out a viral infection – we all got incredibly excited at one point when Ginny read that encephalitis can be caused by shingles, which Alan had recently had. But no. Then a lumbar puncture ruled out a bacterial cause. Who knew that the fluid around your spine is the same as that in your brain? Not me. All the time, we were trying to leap ahead, saying to the doctors, 'Well, if it is this, how will you treat it? And what will the likely outcome be? And how long will it take?' But the doctors will not be rushed, and rightly so. In fact, establishing what they *don't* know is probably just as important as recording what they *do* know.

Unfortunately, the medical profession can sometimes get to the point where there are no more tests they can do and then they will have to give you an assumed diagnosis simply because they have ruled out everything else. This is often the case with illnesses such as ME (myalgic encephalomyelitis) for example, and indeed sometimes with encephalitis. This can be a nightmare for a patient, as many things from sick pay to health insurance can depend on that vital piece of paper confirming exactly what the patient is suffering from. With Alan, we were lucky – lucky by just seven years. Doctors have known since the

1970s that if encephalitis doesn't have a bacterial or viral cause then it could be caused by the body's own immune system malfunctioning and producing antibodies that attack the brain. But the blood test to discover these antibodies wasn't created until 2005. And the test to find the specific antibodies that Alan's immune system was producing (GABA B) wasn't devised until 2010.

Encephalitis: a quick guide

The simple explanation of 'an inflammation of the brain caused by an infection or through the immune system attacking the brain in error' is just the start of understanding this complicated illness, where medical science is still making major advances. Children can get it, adults can get it and, according to the Encephalitis Society, there are up to 6000 cases in the UK each year. Some patients make a complete recovery, some die, most are somewhere in between. The Encephalitis Society say that 'no two people affected will have the same outcome and the effects can be long-term. Nerve cells may be damaged or destroyed and this damage is termed acquired brain injury.' It lists the most common after-effects as 'tiredness, recurring headaches, difficulties with memory, concentration, balance, mood swings, aggression, clumsiness, epilepsy, physical problems, speech and language problems, reduced speed of thought and reaction, changes in personality and in the ability to function day-to-day', which is not a list that makes for cheerful reading. Neither does the fact that in 50% of the cases of Alan's type of encephalitis, the immune system has glitched because it has detected microscopic tumours.

Detached from reality

One day, very early on, I asked Alan if he could say how the encephalitis felt and he said that it seemed as if he was floating in a sphere and that everyone else was in a different sphere. I was so struck by this image that I took out my phone and asked him to describe what it was like again as I recorded it. His exact words were:

> You feel really like you are a wraith completely detached from reality, floating around. But you're also a reality, detached from the wraith. You're not as one person, one being, and everything around you is separate and complete and operating on its own. The most frightening thing about this is that you feel so detached from the core of your life and that you are operating in a sort of separate zone from everyone else with no way of linking in to what they are doing or thinking.

Although it's muddled, I found it extremely revealing. I've never heard Alan say anything like this since.

The problems of unusual illnesses

In the beginning, I thought that an illness caused by your own immune system malfunctioning wasn't likely to be nearly as serious as one caused by a viral or a bacterial infection. How could it possibly be that your own body can produce something that will cause severe brain damage – and in some cases kill you? But I discovered quite quickly that, in fact, your own immune system can be as powerful a force as any germ or virus. As virologist

Dr Chris Smith says, 'the immune system is the most complex organ that we have...it is a very powerful force and when it goes wrong it can unleash devastating damage to whatever it chooses to target'. I also came to realise that Alan was 'lucky' that his encephalitis began with seizures, as it meant he was admitted very swiftly. I read an account by Professor Tom Solomon, one of the UK's experts on encephalitis, which tells me that only half of encephalitis cases start with seizures, and in the other half, 'when patients are just behaving strangely, it is much harder to work out what is going on. Sometimes it is thought the patient is drunk, has taken drugs or that they have a psychiatric illness.'

I still find it frustrating that whenever I tell someone about Alan, the chances are they don't know what I'm talking about. I suspect that everyone who suffers from something unusual has the same problem – it's hard to take something seriously if you've never heard of it. The Encephalitis Society believe that although 500,000 people globally are affected by encephalitis every year, 78% of people don't know what it is.

A cure?

The phrase 'a cure for cancer' is right up there as one of life's goals for idealists along with 'world peace'. I gradually learn that the healthcare system isn't always in the business of 'cures'. What they are hoping to find is a 'treatment' for the illness, which is very different from magically vanishing it away. Having established that the encephalitis is caused by rogue antibodies in Alan's blood, the medical conundrum is how to get rid of them. The two options available are, first, a drug called Rituximab, which will zap them. The second idea is to take all of Alan's blood out, wash it clean of the antibodies and then put it back into him – a process called plasma exchange. These both sound pretty much like miracles, and the doctors confirm that the results can be dramatic. And we are both fortunate and grateful that these expensive and complex options are made available to Alan. But over the months, I discover that the damage an illness has done while it's wreaking havoc in your body can be more relevant to the eventual outcome than any wondrous remedy.

Wanting the world to know

Using the internet as a public documentation of illness is increasingly popular. Starting a blog, tweeting about your progress and creating new Facebook or Instagram accounts are all ways to share your story. And revealing what has happened to you to complete strangers can be a therapeutic and powerful thing to do, bringing benefits to both the patient and the public. Many of us have been hugely moved by some of the extraordinarily brave memoirs written by those who are seriously ill. There is no better way than the web to reach so many people so quickly or so easily. And, unlike a printed book, those reading your story can reach right back to you, straight away. Which, again, can provide much comfort and support.

But, as with all social media, if your sense of self-worth becomes overly dependent on 'likes' or 'views', then what seemed like a good thing can become a bad thing. Raising an army of followers is not going to work for everyone. As well as blogging, using the internet to crowdfund for help with medicines is on the rise, which means telling your story and not just hoping for ♥♥♥ but also £££. For cancer treatments alone, more than £4.5 million was raised by crowdfunding on JustGiving UK in 2016, according to the website's own figures.

The first question has to be whether the 'treatments' on offer actually work. Research by *The BMJ* (2018) finds that 'many people fear that crowdfunding has opened up a new and lucrative revenue stream for cranks, charlatans and conmen who prey on the vulnerable'. But also, I wonder if the supposed support of complete strangers could do more harm than good in the long term for people who are ill.

Jessica Mitchell, who set up a Facebook fundraising campaign to raise money for her son Dylan's cancer treatment, talked to *The Telegraph* about how hard it can be when other parents' campaigns are more successful than yours. 'You don't begrudge them the money, but there's a sort of jealousy. You can't help thinking, why is their child more important than mine?' She also worries about becoming 'almost public property' to those who are kind enough to donate. *The Guardian* quotes an American professor who says, 'crowdfunding is popularising a new sort of economic marketplace, where people are essentially marketing themselves...you need to compete with all these other people to be the most deserving, the most needy, the most compelling'.

A mother in Norfolk told *The Guardian* how she hoped to raise at least £250,000 for experimental cancer treatment. She said that she found comfort from 'the positive feeling that comes from knowing all those people are working so hard to get me the treatment I need'. But what if people aren't 'working so hard'? A London taxi driver trying to raise money via Facebook for his son with leukaemia spoke of his heartbreak over not raising enough. He raised only £18,460 of his £540,000 target and his son died aged 12. 'I felt like people were inhumane. You put in all this effort and then not a lot of people donate.'

And we can all remember the terribly sad story of Charlie Gard, a boy born in August 2016 with a rare genetic disorder, who mobilised enormous public support, thanks in part to the newspapers. His parents raised nearly £1.4 million to try and keep their little boy alive but he died, and you do wonder how much help #CharliesArmy is to his parents now. What happens when the public and the newspapers have moved on to something else and the comfort of strangers has melted away? Is it harder to cope alone after such high levels of interest and involvement?

How doctors break bad news

Christie Watson, in her wonderful book *The Language of Kindness: A Nurse's Story*, says that 'a nurse must judge the character of the family member. If information is given in a way that the family can't comprehend it, all manner of things may go wrong...they can feel cheated or tricked somehow.'

Before Alan got ill, I imagined that it would be obvious when a doctor was going to tell you something bad. I envisaged a solemn face, a hushed voice, possibly a secluded room. Five months of being in hospital every day showed me that it's not like that at all. First, in many hospitals there will be an ever-changing rota and you may never see the same doctor twice. And unless the doctors have written very detailed notes (which they won't), they will never really be aware of who has already told you what.

Second, I think doctors have an unofficial policy of not necessarily telling you what the prognosis is unless you ask, releasing their information on a 'need-to-know' basis. I can see the rationale behind this, but it can be frustrating. I think many patients would rather adopt a 'prepare for the worst, hope for the best' mindset.

Third, even if they have told you something, it's quite likely (especially if it's bad news) that you won't have properly absorbed it. With Alan, since he had no short-term memory and found it extraordinarily hard to process information, anything the doctors told him almost literally went in one ear and out the other. Oddly, although he was on the neurology ward, many doctors seemed to struggle with this fact. Eventually, the message got through that unless I was there to hear it, anything they told Alan was not going to be recalled and was therefore pointless. In fact, I think it is immensely useful for any patient, whatever their ailment, to have someone else there to help process what the doctors are saying.

The problem is that you never know exactly when the doctors are going to impart their most important words of wisdom. On some days our conversations were almost social and then on others I would be bombarded with new facts. The day that Alan's neurology consultant tells me perhaps the worst news of all, there is no preamble and it is revealed just as Izzy and I are about to leave. 'Oh, I'm glad I've caught you,' she says. 'I've got the results of Alan's latest MRI scan.' She's looking at me very intently. 'There's no change,' she says. 'It all looks stable. But we can see that he's always going to have problems with memory and processing.' She pauses and then continues, 'The atrophy on that side of his brain is permanent.' I nod. 'I understand,' I say, although my mind is whirring. She is telling me that Alan will never be the same again, but because the word 'stable' sounds so promising, it takes us both a while to process exactly what she's telling us. Afterwards, outside the hospital, we have a long, long hug.

Go your own way

There is more than one way to do most things, and there is certainly more than one way to cope with illness. For me, one of the strategies has been writing this book. I have reframed what has happened to Alan and our family as a narrative that both we, and hopefully others, can gain something from. I love writing. I like the process of it, and (like my grandmother and my mother) I like to turn things that have happened into stories. I can see that this has been one of my ways of processing what has happened. But it is not for everyone. Susan Sontag, in her seminal book *Illness as Metaphor*, argued strongly that by turning cancer into a foe to be battled rather than an illness to be cured, we are suggesting that patients are the architects of their own fate, which, in many cases, is untrue. I completely understand that. But although you don't have a choice about being ill, you do have a choice in how you deal with it, and remembering that can be empowering.

Ten (equally valid) ways to deal with illness

1. *I'm going to fight it*

Many people want to battle. Every triumph of chemotherapy or surgery is a win to celebrate, every setback, a loss to bounce back from. In many hospitals, it has become common for patients to ring a bell at the end of chemotherapy or radiation to show they have beaten the disease, which is a very public and powerful symbol of victory and celebration.

2. *I'm going to accept it*

Some patients, especially if the illness has been prolonged, make the decision to let things take their course, come what may. This can be extremely upsetting for relatives – I think of Dylan Thomas's famous exhortation to his father not to be passive, but to 'rage, rage against the dying of the light' – but it is a choice that anyone is entitled to make.

3. *I'm going to become an expert*

Researching the hell out of the illness, reading everything that's written about it and investigating a cure can be a way of taking back control. Such is the availability of information, thanks to the internet, that you can soon know more than your doctor does, especially if it is rare. I sometimes think of this as a 'Superman' approach, after Christopher Reeve, the Hollywood actor who in films could only be defeated by kryptonite, but in real life was paralysed in a riding accident. He set up a foundation to fund innovative medical research into spinal cord injuries and never gave up hope that he would walk again. He never did, and he died in 2004, but his foundation has invested over $138 million in research labs around the world.

4. *I'm going to help others*

'Is there anything I can do?' is the question asked by both patients given a grim diagnosis and their families, who just want to do something. And yes, there is, thanks to the hundreds of charities both large and small that will embrace your assistance with open arms. Getting involved on any level – from donations, to running marathons, to baking cakes, to hosting tea parties – will make a genuine difference. And throwing yourself altruistically into benefitting others can reduce the horrible helplessness that is often the unwelcome companion to injury and illness. Lucy ran 10K in 2019 and raised money on behalf of the Encephalitis Society. It was undoubtably a powerful motivation for her to help others struck down by the thing that she had seen affect her dad.

5. I'm going to ignore it

In Raynor Winn's powerful book *The Salt Path*, she describes how she felt when the doctor told her that her husband Moth had a terminal, degenerative illness. 'I hated the doctor, sitting on the edge of his desk delivering his diagnosis as if he was presenting a gift. The best thing I can do for you, Moth, is give you a diagnosis. It was the very worst thing he could do. I wished he could take it away and let me live without knowing. I didn't want to see the black void of my future every time I looked at Moth.' Raynor and Moth decide to ignore the doctor's prognosis and walk the 630-mile South West Coast Path. It wouldn't suit everyone, but it was undeniably the right decision for them.

6. I'm going to share it

Even in my lifetime, the progress that has been made in talking about medical matters is staggering. I can remember a time not so very long ago, when most people, both on TV and in general, wouldn't talk about breast cancer, purely because they didn't feel comfortable saying the word 'breast'. No one ever said words like 'hysterectomy', 'prostate' or 'cervical' without lowering their voices and looking furtive. And, of course, mental health issues were totally taboo, with 'baby blues', 'his nerves' or 'her condition' pretty much universally used. Every time we talk openly, we are raising awareness and, in the cases of illnesses where prompt treatment is vital, saving lives. Jade Goody talking about cervical cancer, Lena Dunham about endometriosis, Michael J. Fox about Parkinson's, Charlie Sheen about HIV and Michael Phelps about depression are examples of famous people who have helped others by sharing, and of course there are many more.

7. I'm keeping it to myself

But for some people, for everyone to know is a devastating invasion of privacy that is not remotely helpful. There will always be a friend to tell you that you shouldn't 'bottle things up', but for some, 'holding it all together' rather than telling lots of other people, which would make you feel vulnerable and exposed, is a valid strategy. You are totally entitled to keep your own illness a secret if you want to.

8. I'm taking one day at a time

When Alan first fell ill, I found one of the most useful things of all was not to look too far ahead. Shrinking the timescale so that I just focused on getting through each day really made things easier. It was a big challenge to change my thinking, as I'm a person who usually likes to look forward and hypothesise about possible scenarios. King Solomon, when asked by his subjects for a phrase that would be true in any situation, said, 'This too shall pass away.' Numerous people have found this motto useful in times of hardship, to remind them that even great suffering cannot last forever. (Of course, it can also serve as a reminder to savour the good times, as joy is also transient.)

9. I'm searching for the hero inside myself

Deciding that you are the star of your own story, rather than a victim, can give you extra strength. If you feel that no one understands what you are going through, you can change that by writing or recording exactly how you feel. No one can challenge your own emotions; the narrative is yours to tell as you want, and doing this can be empowering.

10. I'm muddling through

In other words, don't overthink what has happened, just get on with it. As John Lennon famously said, 'Life is what happens to you while you're busy making other plans.' Carrying on with as much normal stuff as possible, not making a drama at any point and just seeing how things pan out is probably the most common strategy of all, and 'keeping on keeping on' suits lots of us just fine.

Chapter Five

HOSPITAL HACKS

The Practical Stuff

'The thing is, I really don't like hospitals'

THE SECOND MOST COMMON expression after 'I can't believe this is happening to me' is 'I don't like hospitals.' It's extraordinary how often you hear that phrase, from visitors, relations, other patients, absolutely everyone in fact, apart from the 1.5 million staff in the UK who work for the NHS and maybe they're not always that keen either! Things we especially don't like include: the smell of death, the smell of bleach, the squeaky floors, the silent doors, the quiet corridors and the noisy wards. Also, the machines, the needles, the bins, the blue curtains and the beds. It's often said almost conspiratorially, as if imparting a great secret. A kind of 'Shh, don't tell anyone, but I don't like hospitals.' A would-be visitor will say apologetically, 'Oh of course I'd love to come in and see him, but the thing is, I really don't like hospitals.' Another person on the ward will tell you, 'It's particularly hard you see, because she really doesn't like hospitals.' I get it, I really do: hospitals remind us of our own mortality and of deeply stressful times, but do you really think that there's a bunch of people bouncing around shouting, 'Oh goodie, a hospital!'? Perhaps every hospital ought to have a large sign above the entrance that reads: NO ONE LIKES HOSPITALS! GET OVER YOURSELF!

However, there are lots of tips and tricks I've learnt from spending so much time in hospitals, which I hope will make things a little bit easier.

A special relationship?

Building a relationship with a doctor is a bizarre experience. We want doctors to like us, and we want to like them. Straight away, we want them to be much more interested in us than is realistic. We know it's selfish, but we want them to prioritise our care or the care of those who matter to us. And we want them to mind about us and not to be too busy. Adam Kay, author of the hilarious *This is Going to Hurt: Secret Diaries of a Junior Doctor*, says 'Just remember that a doctor is someone with a flat and a partner and a life,'[1] and we'd say 'Right back at ya Adam, just remember that we too have complex and varied lives, there's more going on with us than just this crappy illness you know.' For many of us, a conversation with a doctor will be one of the most meaningful and memorable moments of our lives. But for the doctors, it is just another day at work, which means there is almost bound to be a sharp discrepancy between expectations and outcomes.

---

1   Reproduced from *This is Going to Hurt* by Adam Kay (copyright © Adam Kay 2017) with permission from Pan Macmillan through PLSclear.

The dos and don'ts of how to talk and listen to doctors

- Do record the conversation on your phone and then you can play it back to yourself later.
- Do take a friend.
- Don't decide you don't like them. This is entirely counterproductive.
- Do carry a short summary of your previous medical conditions. It's often easier to give this to a new doctor than stammering through an explanation.
- Don't have preconceived ideas about the solution.
- Do listen – and ask a doctor to repeat something if you need to.
- Do ask questions. Doctors are happier with stats than guesswork. For example, 'What percentage of patients with my type of cancer survive?' is more likely to get an accurate answer than 'How long have I got?'
- Do make your questions personal and direct. Rather than saying 'But what happens if the medicine doesn't work?', say 'What should I do if I still have a high temperature tomorrow?'
- Don't think that a doctor with poor personal skills is necessarily a bad doctor.

Crossed wires

During Alan's stay, he frequently needs to be taken to another part of the hospital for a scan or other procedure. And here I discover that the communication between the different parts of the hospital is appalling. Scans are scheduled and then missed because no one has told the ward. Porters wheel him to entirely random departments, bemused doctors send him back, sometimes nurses accompany him, but notes are left behind. And all the time things are muddled further by the fact that Alan himself doesn't know where he is, a fact that doesn't seem to be fully factored in by the staff as he is moved around the labyrinthine corridors.

Once he is travelling between hospitals in taxis, things are even more chaotic and are often made worse by doctors' dreadful handwriting. On one occasion, I meet him at the reception desk of a hospital that we've never been to before, where he has been taken for a scan. The nurse who accompanies him has only brought a scruffy piece of paper with a name scribbled on it in pencil. It is so poorly misspelled that the reception staff genuinely have no idea where he should go, and it is only because I am there to decipher the note that he ends up where he is supposed to be.

Communication issues seem to run throughout the healthcare system. Just the other day, I was speaking to a social worker on the phone who was checking the emergency contacts she had for Alan. She told me she had 'Gin and Gary' written on her form by a colleague. 'Is that two friends?' she asked. I was utterly bewildered until I realised that what it should say was 'Ginny Curry' – Alan's sister! Even Alan's own neurologist has almost illegible writing, and whenever she scribbles his next appointment time on the booking form, I wonder why she can't take half a second longer to write it properly. I know it's a cliché that doctors have poor handwriting; but really, why?

My advice would be never to assume that any doctor or nurse has necessarily passed all the information on to their colleagues correctly. Keep copies of all letters (take photos on your phone), ask exactly where doctors are sending you to if it's another department or hospital, watch while they are writing notes and, if necessary, ask what they're recommending and write it down yourself! It is also completely fine if you don't catch a doctor or nurse's name to ask them to spell it for you, so you know exactly who you have been speaking to.

The lifts

Another thing that people really don't like is lifts. And hospital lifts surely fall into a special hellish category of their own. Claustrophobic and germ ridden at the best of times, they are far from ideal in a situation where most people are already either a) stressed or b) ill. However, there is no avoiding them, Alan's ward is on the tenth floor. We soon discover that the lifts in our hospital are so notorious that they should have their own Facebook page. In theory, there are five of them, but at least one and often two are always out of order. And they are situated on adjacent sides of a corner, so you need to press two separate buttons to summon them and then keep dodging back and forth to see which one comes first. If there's an enormous queue, obviously this behaviour is not acceptable, so you join a waiting group and then listen to other lifts arriving while wondering why yours appears to be stuck on floor 15.

Once you are in a lift, your tribulations are not over. It will stop on every single floor. And on every floor the doors will open. Sometimes, a very large or very frail person at the back of your lift will attempt to push their way out. Nobody wants to leave the lift to make this easier, for fear that they will not get back in again. Sometimes there will be a person in a wheelchair waiting to get into the packed lift. There will be a long moment where they gaze at you mournfully and you will all stare sympathetically but resolutely back. They will then sigh and say, 'I guess I'll get the next one then,' and you will all nod with a little smile of pretend regret but really unreserved relief that you are the one in the lift and not the wheelchair. Someone will say, 'I'm sure it won't be long,' while you are all thinking, 'Actually, you are probably going to die waiting.' Sometimes the doors will open and there will be no one there at all. This feels strangely spooky, as if a person has just been vaporised. It is quite likely that someone will actually sing *The Twilight Zone* music. The lift will then sit there, doors gaping, going nowhere. An impatient man will then bellow, 'Press the *Doors Close* button!' A flustered woman will then accidentally press the *Doors Open* button, which means the lift will decide to have a little sulk and you will not be going anywhere for another four hours. On one occasion, the lift lurched and clunked its way up in such an alarming manner that we collectively decided to get out on floor 6, and there was then a surreal moment where 12 strangers all looked at each other and said 'Where the hell are we?' before bonding while trying to find our way to another floor, like the end of a disaster movie.

All of these shenanigans mean that ascending to visit Alan on the tenth floor can take at least ten minutes. That also means that if you are up in the ward and decide to go and get a cup of tea or a newspaper, or put some money in the parking meter, you will be genuinely lucky if you are back within 20 minutes. However, eventually we learn a little trick. There is an express lift, specially designed to whisk people to floor 11, which is where the wards for private patients are located. It stops just once on the way up, so it takes a fraction of the time. And therefore, the genius plan of getting this lift to floor 11 and then walking down one flight of stairs to the tenth must have saved us hours.

The two tips I would offer to anyone visiting a hospital with lifts are these. First, allow a lot of extra time to get to your appointment. I witnessed far too many people in a state of genuine anxiety because the lifts were going to make them late. Second, if you are only going to the first floor, *you can definitely walk!* This will free up the lifts and will be good for you and everyone else! Maybe you are thinking, well why didn't *you* walk up the stairs to the tenth floor then? Good question, and my sprightlier sister Alice did successfully achieve this. However, the one time I attempted it, Sam and I only got to the fifth floor before I had to admit defeat after becoming a sweaty wheezing mess. Sam, of course, was stepping onwards and upwards.

The dangers of Google: proceed with caution

'I think it's encephalitis,' says the bald and brainy neurologist. My first reaction, even though I don't say it, is 'Encepha...what? Can you please talk English? There must be a simpler explanation – ordinary people like us just don't get weird illnesses that no one's ever heard of.' Afterwards, it reminded me of the time when Sam was about five and had an odd rash on his side. I took him to the doctor, and she said, 'Ah yes, what we have here is molluscum contagiosum.' It sounded so like something out of *Harry Potter* that I honestly thought she was making a peculiar medical joke and laughed out loud, waiting for her to tell me what it really was. Then I realised that she wasn't joking, and yes, this common childhood skin complaint really did have a silly Latin name.

Back to the neurologist, and to be fair, he immediately follows up by telling me that encephalitis means Alan's brain is inflamed and there are various reasons why this could happen. These days, I sometimes say to people that encephalitis is 'a bit like meningitis' because more people have heard of that – they know it's to do with your brain and they know it's serious. But often, your first reaction when you hear something you don't understand is to Google it. When the neurologist said 'encephalitis' I wanted to know as much as he could tell me and, like most people, I've never felt as if any doctor has had quite as much time to explain things to me as I'd have liked. But once I was back home, I didn't Google it. I was too frightened of what I might discover. I was right to be wary; other family members did Google encephalitis and told me afterwards that it was extremely scary.

The fact is, finding out more wasn't going to help Alan. It is highly unlikely that an amateur search is going to uncover something the professionals don't know and, by trying to, you may well terrify yourself in the process.

To try to make Alan better, the doctors moved forward one small step at a time, and the internet doesn't do that: it takes a giant leap into all of the information. And it is not your friend. I mean that quite literally: it will not impart knowledge to you caringly, slowly, thoughtfully. It will give it to you bluntly, graphically and – often – incorrectly. I once saw a cartoon of a GP sitting in his surgery wearing a T-shirt that says 'Don't confuse your Google search with my medical degree', and I think this is a good message to keep in mind. Doctors are sometimes criticised for the way they impart information to patients, and many have a far from perfect 'bedside manner'. But even the most abrupt professional has more empathy than a search engine.

I have come to realise that doctors are usually trying to assess the level of information that they think you can cope with and then impart it accordingly. This can be infuriating, and sometimes patients feel like shouting 'Give me the facts' or 'Tell it to me straight.' Assessing what each person does or doesn't want to know – and perhaps even more relevantly, what each patient is capable of understanding – is tricky. But doctors are at least trying to get this right in a way that the internet isn't. Google doesn't care whether the information it's giving you is kind or cruel, right or wrong. And because of the way its algorithm works, it will give you the most 'popular' information first. In the case of illness, 'popular' can mean newsworthy, grisly, sensationalist or even downright inaccurate. Sitting in front of a computer screen is a lonely place to be and I would be extremely cautious about 'doing your own research'. If you want to know more than your doctor is telling you, I recommend that you get your information, at least in the early days, in a more curated form, such as from the NHS website, a charity's leaflet or a book.

An apple a day keeps the doctor away?

I discover that Alan is asked each day to choose his food from a staggeringly long menu, and unless I am there to help him, this results in a diet that is far from nutritious. There are so many issues that it's hard to know where to start, but the main ones are that he will pick the same thing every day, he will not add any vegetables to his meal and he will not include the healthy additions that he is 'allowed' such as a yogurt, a piece of fruit or a glass of orange juice. In Alan's case, this is simply because his brain can't 'do' choice, but for other patients, it might be that they are actively opting to eat unhealthily. Without my assistance, every day Alan would eat: cornflakes, white toast, macaroni cheese, cake and custard, macaroni cheese, crumble and custard.

The government announced a review of hospital food in August 2019, saying that 'every year, the NHS serves more than 140 million meals to patients across the country. The quality and nutritional value of these meals can vary substantially.' Boris Johnson agreed that 'guaranteeing hospitals serve nutritional, tasty and fresh meals will not only aid patient recovery, but also fuel staff and visitors.' The healthy-diet advice from the World Health Organization is to include plenty of vegetables, fruit, lentils, beans, nuts and whole grains, and not much salt, sugar and saturated/trans fats. Even a cursory glance at what is served both to patients and in hospital cafés reveals that this guidance is not followed. The rules on what food visitors are allowed to bring in varies enormously between both wards and hospitals, and it is hard to supplement a patient's diet in any useful way. It is a tricky one, as I know all too well that if you are feeling stressed and wrung out, you feel like a slice of cake and a cup of tea, not an apple and a glass of water. We want comforting, but we don't want junk. We want nutritious and wholesome, but we don't want unappealing and boring. I think one solution would be for hospitals to offer far less choice but ensure that the food they do serve is fresher and better.

Nighty-night, sleep tight?

One of the absolute cornerstones of wellbeing is sleep. Sleep expert Mathew Walker argues that it is more important for our health than diet or exercise. Many of the factors that affect sleep at home – not being active, too little fresh air, worry, a noisy room, too hot, too cold, artificial light, boredom, anxiety, other people snoring – are magnified in hospital, and sleeping properly on a ward can be extremely difficult. However, Alan had no issues with sleeping. His problem was that if he left his bed to go to the loo, he couldn't remember which bed to get back into! Once I arrived on the ward to find him napping in the bed of a chap who had been taken off for a scan. Fortunately, I managed to wake him up and move him before the other man returned! Even now, he has the same problem at home. Despite having slept in the same double bed for the 27 years we've been married, he can still 'get lost' in the four metres between the bathroom and the bedroom. One afternoon, we found him happily slumbering in Sam's top bunk bed!

Ten things that may help you to sleep in hospital

- Wearing an eye mask. Even though the lights are dimmed at night-time, many people find a ward has too much light to be able to sleep properly. An eye mask can be a big help.
- Putting on headphones. Wards can be noisy, and playing soft music from your phone or ambient sounds like waves or birdsong can be a good way to block out the bloke grunting in the bed next to you.
- Getting outside. Everyone sleeps better if they've had some fresh air. And living in an air-conditioned or overheated atmosphere for days on end is not conducive to a good night's kip. If you are visiting,

helping someone to get outside just for ten minutes can be a real kindness. You might have to find a wheelchair to take them in, but most hospitals have an unofficial procedure to enable smokers to get outside and there's no reason why non-smokers shouldn't be afforded the same freedom.

- Looking out of a window. Even if a patient can't go outside, being able to see daylight is vitally important to our body's circadian rhythms. Days spent in purely artificial light are known to disrupt our sleep patterns, so try and spend some time near a source of natural light. Again, if you are a visitor, walking over to a window with a patient is a good idea.
- Extra blankets. Hospitals are warm, and patients usually only need one light blanket. However, there are plenty of studies that show that having a heavier blanket can help you sleep better. The snuggly, swaddled feeling has a similar effect to being hugged and can lower your heart rate. The gentle pressure has also been found to increase serotonin, a neurotransmitter involved in sleep regulation, and it encourages your body to produce oxytocin, which can make you feel calmer. You can ask a nurse to give you some extra blankets or bring in your own.
- Bed socks. A 2007 study reported that adults who wore socks in bed got to sleep faster and, anecdotally, most of us find that it is hard to get to sleep if your feet are cold! Many hospitals will give patients regulation NHS slipper socks, but be aware that if

you are bringing in your own, they must have a tread so that they are non-slip/non-skid.

- A scented pillow. The smell in hospitals can be an unpleasant mix of the unfamiliar, the overly clinical and worse. Spraying a lavender linen spray onto your pillow might be a good way of helping you drift off. Research confirms that lavender oil has a sedative effect, lowering the heart rate and reducing anxiety.
- Listening to a story. Audio books that you can download on your phone are not expensive, and lots of people find that listening to a soothing voice is soporific.
- Reading a story. A printed book rather than one on a screen is much better for your eyes at bedtime, and a few pages of a familiar favourite can be a good way to nod off.
- A warm milky drink. The times of day that hospitals serve food and drinks can be problematic for patients' sleep patterns. The last meal of the day is often served far earlier than you might be used to, and it is sometimes followed by a cup of tea or coffee, which is not ideal for those who find that caffeine affects their sleep. A warm drink can help you drop off, but the chances of this being available when you want it are slim. If you are visiting someone, bringing them an insulated cup or small thermos of something like hot chocolate or milky decaffeinated coffee, which they can drink when they want to, could be really helpful.

The many tribulations of hospital parking

The issue of parking at hospitals is a highly contentious one. Like a lot of hospital problems, the true difficulties of the situation only become clear once you are right in the middle of them.

The first hospital Alan is in has a large car park, but in fact it is not large enough, so if you arrive in the afternoon, it is totally full and you must drive round and round hoping that someone will leave. And it is expensive. The second hospital has no car park at all, so street parking is the only option, which is hard to find and costs a fortune and, of course, you need the right money for the meter.

In 2018, the *Express* ran a tragic story about a man who spent hours trying to park at a hospital because he did not have any spare change and then died of a massive aneurysm. The *Mirror* in 2019 claimed that 'cash-strapped families with seriously ill children were forced to spend at least £5 million last year on travel to and from hospitals and families are being pushed into spiralling debt' and told the story of a woman who had spent thousands of pounds on parking since her daughter was diagnosed with cancer. *The Guardian* informs me that, in 2017–18, English NHS trusts made more than £226 million from car parks.

There are clearly some unavoidable issues. Hospitals in cities only have a limited amount of space and there often isn't room to enlarge the car parks as hospitals expand. Street parking around a hospital frequently needs to be regulated in order to avoid a total nightmare for residents. If a hospital is next to a station, it is likely that any free parking will be nabbed by commuters, meaning that visitors have nowhere to go.

Car parks have been free in hospitals in Scotland and Wales since 2008 (the year before this, Welsh hospitals collected nearly

£5.4 million in charges, which, when you bear in mind that only three million people live in Wales, is pretty extraordinary) with the payments labelled as a 'tax on the sick' by the British Medical Association. But a free car park usually seems to mean an overflowing car park. An investigation by *The Sunday Post* (2013) found that a lack of parking space was costing NHS Scotland millions of pounds in missed appointments.

Daniel Pryor writing for the Adam Smith Institute (2017) argues the case against free hospital parking, saying 'spending money on this means not spending that money elsewhere' and that 'I'd be very surprised if local health trusts viewed free parking as a better use of £200 million than spending more on frontline care, mental health services, or any number of other options'. He believes that 'most Brits (begrudgingly) accept that there are a small number of things (like prescription charges) that aren't free on the NHS for common-sense, practical reasons. Hospital car park charges firmly belong in this category.' A private members' bill to abolish hospital parking charges in England tried and failed to get through parliament in 2018.

I don't know what the answer is. Some hospitals provide free or discounted parking for certain groups, such as disabled people and staff, and personally, I feel that this group should also include those with seriously ill children and people on a low income.

When Alan first went into hospital, on most days I arrived in the morning and didn't leave until the evening. Once, after an incredibly long and stressful day, my little Nissan Micra was the last car left in the car park. Under the lamplight in the dark, driving rain it looked as solitary and lonely as I felt, and I was so upset by the day's events that for a long while I couldn't remember where I put my parking ticket. The thought of walking back across the huge car park and trying to find someone to help me or paying the large fine for having a lost ticket was horrible, and by the time I finally found the ticket I was crying. There must be hundreds of people having similar experiences every day.

After a week or so in the hospital, one of the nurses mentions almost casually that a discount on the parking is available for long-term visitors. She finds me a form, which I duly fill in. The system is complicated and a bit haphazard. Once a week, I must take the form to a small porters' office behind reception, which is frequently unstaffed. They tell me there that I can park in the maternity ward car park, which is a bit cheaper, and give me a special code. It all seems a bit dodgy and, as with a lot of hospital systems, it seems as if I have found out about it by accident.

Parking tips

- Get a friend to drop you off and pick you up. People often ask if there's anything they can do to help you, and this is incredibly useful.
- Consider parking about a ten-minute walk away if you can. You will need more time of course, but a walk at the start and end of a visit can help clear your head.
- Download a parking app such as RingGo, PayBy-Phone, ParkRight or AppyParking on your phone. The big advantage of these apps is that you can pay without physically using a card or coins and can top up the time while you are inside the hospital, so you don't have to run outside to feed the meter.
- Set an alarm on your phone to go off ten minutes before your parking expires.

> • Ask if there are parking discounts available for long-term patients/visitors. No one will think to tell you this.

Sort it out

When you are plunged into the world of long-term illness, life seems to stop. But, of course, it doesn't. In the weeks after Alan went into hospital, I was in a total daze, but my family still needed to be fed, the dog walked, the work done, the bills paid. In the early days, I recommend making a 'to-do' list and then asking a friend or family member to help you go through it, prioritising what is and isn't important. You might be surprised by someone else's perspective on what you do and don't need to do.

For me, the first decision was to contact the client who had offered me a writing job at the start of the year and turn it down. I just wasn't going to have the time or headspace, and making that decision quickly, rather than struggling on, saved me a lot of worry. Don't take on more than you can cope with and put yourself under too much pressure. I would also prioritise paying bills on time and dealing with other unpleasant tasks, even if you are usually the sort of person who leaves a pile of paperwork to mount up. Getting on top of things you *can* control will often help you feel better about the things you can't.

And if you want to provide real help for a pal, find a way to help them clean their house! There is nothing more soul destroying than coming back to a grubby, messy home after a long day in a hospital.

What you need to take on board when someone you love

is taken into hospital is that it is not just the hospital staff who are in 'emergency mode', it's you too. They are using specialist staff and resources, and you should feel entitled to do exactly the same. So, don't think 'Oh well, I'll just muddle along' when your whole life has been turned upside down; draft in as much specialist help as you need and can afford.

The hell of A&E

Alan's journey through the hospital system began in an ambulance, but for many people it starts in A&E. Just before the general election in December 2019, hospitals hit the headlines for the zillionth time when Boris Johnson refused to look at a picture of a small boy sleeping on a pile of coats in the A&E department of the Leeds General Infirmary. A surprising aspect of the story was that this was not a child who had been brought in by his parents but a little boy who was brought in by paramedics. I think many people are under the misapprehension that if you are ill enough to need an ambulance, you will somehow skip the A&E department, but this is not always the case.

Emergency departments are all slightly different, but the procedure is generally that you will be seen by a number of different professionals, with long waits in between each stage. You will begin with a receptionist, move on to what is sometimes described as a triage nurse, who will make an initial assessment, and after that you may see a doctor or nurse. You may be treated, you may be sent home, you may be allocated a bed on the emergency ward or maybe even admitted. Where, when and for how long you wait will depend on the seriousness of your case, but it will also have a lot to do with the size of the hospital and how busy it is.

The other factor is that although you are gradually 'moving up the queue', it almost certainly won't feel like it, because the places you are told to wait in do not appear to be in a logical order. In my experience, these have been: a waiting room, a corridor, some random chairs in a hallway, just inside the ambulance loading bay, a mysteriously numbered section (e.g., Area 15C), a foyer, on a bed, on a stretcher. There will be no indication of progression, which for most people (especially in Britain where we like an orderly queue) is stressful.

So you may start off in a half-empty waiting room, then move to some chairs outside a little office, then have a blood test inside the little office, then move to a curtained cubicle, lie down on a bed, be seen by a doctor and feel as if you are getting somewhere, then be told to return to the waiting room, which is now full to overflowing, so you have to stand outside it, next to the toilets where you can no longer hear your name being called. Which definitely feels as if you are going backwards. And all the time there is the nagging feeling that someone else has 'bumped' ahead of you or your notes have fallen out of one of the overflowing wire baskets you have noticed. There is absolutely no way of finding out whereabouts you are in 'the system' without asking one of the harassed nurses. Which you feel very guilty about, as your query takes them away from what they are supposed to be doing and implies that you are hassling them to move you up the queue. Which you are not, you just want some reassurance that you haven't been completely forgotten about and maybe an indication as to how much longer you will be there.

I honestly think you should approach a trip to A&E as if you are about to embark on a long and difficult journey and prepare accordingly. The other factor to bear in mind is that to navigate

A&E alone, with children or with someone who is mentally ill is ten times harder.

An A&E checklist

- A summary of your medical history
- Phone
- Phone charger cable
- Portable charger
- Headphones and music
- Blanket or large scarf
- Some cash (hospital shops don't always take card payments for small amounts)
- A book
- Hand sanitiser
- Water
- A snack
- Wipes
- Another person

Chapter Six

HOW IT
ALL WORKS

The Mechanics of a Hospital

'What are you saying exactly, doctor?'

CO-AUTHOR OF THE BRITISH Medical Association's hand-book on medical ethics, Julian Sheather, writes that 'patients can feel lost in the hyper-specialised fields of modern medicine, their experience of illness dissolved in the arcane language of bio-chemical science', and it is true that one of the most over-whelming parts of a hospital experience is the confusion you can feel whenever a doctor tells you something. Just when you want things to be crystal clear, a word appears that is either totally unfamiliar or looms larger than it should in the conversation, because you only half understand it and it sounds deeply scary.

In 2018, new guidance from the Academy of Medical Royal Colleges set out a series of steps to try and make information less confusing for patients. One piece of advice was that doctors should use 'plain English' where possible, rather than 'confusing medical terms or Latin'. Nevertheless, much of the communication from doctors is still incomprehensible. For me, some of the most alarming words were sepsis, psychosis, nil by mouth, invasive and oedema. Simple explanations of all these and many more can be found in Appendix One: A Medical Jargon Buster.

The words specific to your own illness will take a while to get your head around, and you will then find that you spend an inordinate amount explaining what they mean to friends and family forever after. Our key new words were *confabulation* and *cognitive fatigue*.

Confabulation is a rather wonderful word that means 'the production of fabricated, distorted, or misinterpreted memories about oneself or the world, without the conscious intention to deceive' (Fotopoulou, Conway and Solms, 2007). It occurs after a brain injury or illness and is quite rare. The neurological explanation for exactly what's going on is still contested, but the simplest explanation is that the brain is trying to fill in the blanks. The crucial thing is that a person who confabulates has no idea they are doing it and isn't doing it deliberately. They are also totally unconcerned when you point out the inconsistencies in what they are saying. Sometimes the confabulations are based on real memories, but sometimes they are triggered by entirely random thoughts. So, Alan sometimes thought he'd been in an aeroplane (because his ward was on the tenth floor?) or to the Caribbean (because it was warm?) or to Australia (because the radiologist had an Aussie accent?), but often it was impossible to work out where the 'memories' were coming from. As he got better, the confabulations became more rooted in reality but equally wrong. He is still sometimes adamant that he has just returned from a drive or the office, even though it is over four years since he has done either. He is much more likely to confabulate when he is tired, which brings me to the second issue.

Most people would know that fatigue meant tiredness. But the sort of tiredness you get after a brain injury is entirely different to normal exhaustion. When he needs to rest, Alan's brain simply stops working properly, like a computer trying to shut down. In practical terms, this can mean that he doesn't have enough energy to walk any further for example, but the more usual effects are that he starts confabulating. The only solution is rest. Even nowadays, Alan still needs a huge amount of sleep – two hour-long naps a day and 11 hours at night.

'They're doing some tests'

Everyone who's been into hospital is familiar with this phrase, and a bit of research reveals that, during 2018–19, 23 million diagnostic tests were performed in England's hospitals.

Until the 1950s, all tests were carried out by hand by hospital lab technicians. They were slow and expensive and, of course, sometimes mistakes were made. Automated machines revolutionised the process, and one of the first was the AutoAnalyzer, invented and built in 1951 by Leonard Skeggs, which was a mechanical device able to perform one blood test per minute. There was also the Robot Chemist invented by Hans Baruch (first sold commercially in 1959), which could measure the levels of different chemicals in samples and was probably the first test to use a digital printout for results. More automated lab machines were developed from the 1960s onwards, and developments in robotics and computers meant machines became better and faster. By the end of the 20th century, the tests carried out by the laboratory were central to the workings of a hospital.

Persian physician and philosopher Avicenna said that 'an ignorant doctor is the aide-de-camp of death', and 2000 years later, tests are one of the biggest contributors to making an accurate diagnosis. But what are they all for?

Blood is thicker than water

The Ancient Greeks back in 500 BC knew that blood moved round the body, they knew that there was a difference between the blood carried in veins and that carried in arteries, they knew that blood coagulated and they speculated about the idea of using blood transfusions to save life. The Greek word for blood is 'hema' as in haematology, which is the medical name for the study of blood.

But it wasn't until 1628 that an English physician named William Harvey properly discovered how blood circulated. The first successful blood transfusion was recorded in 1665 by another English doctor, Richard Lower, who transfused blood from one dog to another (with both surviving!). A real breakthrough came in 1901 when Karl Landsteiner, an Austrian scientist, discovered the three human blood groups – A, B and O – and was subsequently awarded the Nobel Prize for medicine. Another important blood-related discovery was the test developed by British immunologist Robert Coombs in 1945 to detect antibodies. Today, those tiny vials can be used to diagnose a huge number of things, and more tests are being developed all the time.

Blood tests can detect...

- Whether any bacteria are present – to check for the presence of an infection.
- Your cholesterol levels – high levels could put you at risk of heart attacks or heart disease.
- The levels of haemoglobin – which carries oxygen from your lungs to the rest of your body.
- The levels of glucose – to diagnose and monitor diabetes.
- Your blood type – essential if you need a transfusion.
- The levels of electrolytes – low levels could indicate dehydration or diabetes.
- A high concentration of proteins – which can indicate inflammation.
- The types and numbers of red blood cells, white blood cells and platelets – which can detect anaemia, infection or inflammation.
- The level of enzymes – which can help to diagnose certain liver conditions, including hepatitis and cirrhosis.
- The presence of certain antibodies. One such test was to prove absolutely crucial in Alan's case, and that particular test was only developed in 2010, which shows how very cutting edge the science of blood testing can be.

Other tests and scans

You may well be sent to another part of a hospital for a scan or test. You will discover that every department believes that theirs is the most efficient and that their colleagues in other areas of the hospital are all incompetent. You will meet consultants, doctors, housekeepers, medical students, nurses, occupational therapists, physiotherapists, porters, radiologists, radiographers, registrars, support workers, technicians and more. There will be those you like and those you don't. You will discover that porters are bolshy to nurses and kind to patients, that nurses are better at injections and blood tests than doctors and that housekeepers are faster at getting things done than doctors or nurses.

Biopsy

The doctors take a tiny sample of tissue from your body to examine it. They will usually do this if they have already detected an abnormality and want to investigate further. This could mean that a part of your body doesn't seem to be working properly, like your kidneys or your liver, or it could be because of some sort of structural change, such as a swelling or a lump.

Blood pressure

Blood pressure describes the strength with which your blood pushes on the sides of your arteries as it's pumped around your body. High blood pressure (hypertension) can put a strain on your arteries and organs, which can increase your risk of having a heart attack or stroke. Low blood pressure (hypotension) isn't usually as serious, although it can cause dizziness. It's measured in millimetres of mercury and given as two figures: the top one is called 'systolic', which means the pressure when your heart pushes blood out, the bottom is called 'diastolic', which is the pressure when your heart rests between beats. Normal blood pressure is between 90/60 and 120/80.

Colonoscopy

This test is used to look for problems in the rectum or colon, such as cancer. During it, a doctor inserts into your bottom a very small tube that has a tiny camera lens at the end, as well as a light. The images are displayed on a computer screen for the doctor to see.

CT scan

A computerised tomography (CT) scan uses X-rays and a computer to create detailed images of the inside of the body, including the internal organs, blood vessels and bones. CT scans are sometimes referred to as CAT scans. They can be used to diagnose all sorts of things, from damage to bones and organs, to strokes and cancer.

ECG

An electrocardiogram (ECG) is used to check your heart's rhythm and electrical activity. Little sticky pads with sensors in are attached to your skin and they pick up the electrical signals produced by your heart each time it beats. These signals are recorded by a machine to see if they're unusual. An ECG can be used to detect:

- arrhythmias: where the heart beats too slowly, too quickly or irregularly

- coronary heart disease and heart attacks: where the heart's blood supply is blocked

- cardiomyopathy: where the heart walls become thickened or enlarged.

Echocardiogram

This is a type of ultrasound that looks at the structure of your heart. While you're lying down, several small sticky electrodes are attached to your chest and connected to a machine that monitors your heart rhythm during the test. A lubricating gel is applied, and an ultrasound probe is then moved over your chest. The small probe sends out high-frequency sound waves that create echoes when they bounce off different parts of the body. These echoes are picked up by the probe and turned into a moving image that's displayed on a monitor.

Laparoscopy

This is a surgical procedure that allows a surgeon to access the inside of your tummy or pelvis through very small incisions. The surgeon will use a tiny camera to help diagnose a wide range of conditions. It can also be used to carry out surgical procedures or take a tissue sample for further testing.

Lumbar puncture

A lumbar puncture (LP), also known as a spinal tap, is where a thin needle is inserted between the bones in your lower spine (under local anaesthetic) to collect a sample of the fluid that is found there. The same fluid is in your spinal canal and your brain, so examining it can help diagnose diseases of the central nervous system. It shouldn't be painful, but you may have a headache and some back pain for a few days afterwards.

Mammogram

A mammogram is a type of breast X-ray and is intended to find tumours or cysts that could be signs of breast cancer. Mammograms are an excellent diagnostic test because they can identify tiny lumps long before they become a problem and long before either you or a doctor would be able to find them by yourself.

MRI scan

An MRI scanner costs around £2 million and, wow, does it look like it! In the early weeks, getting an MRI scan acquired an almost mythical status, like finding, and then drinking from, the holy grail. Eventually, having an MRI scan becomes almost routine, but nevertheless, every time Alan's neurologist says, 'I'll order an MRI, just to check everything is stable,' I remember the long wait we had, our belief in this miracle machine that could see inside Alan's brain and how we hoped that its power would solve everything.

The huge scanner stands inside its own dimly lit room behind a door covered with scary symbols and warnings. The technicians controlling it sit behind a window, speaking to the patient via intercom. It resembles a giant metal doughnut, into which the patient slides, on a narrow hard stretcher. It is like something out of a Stanley Kubrick film, and you do not have to have watched much sci-fi to feel apprehensive. You are not totally enclosed, as the tunnel is open at both ends where your head and feet are, but it can feel somewhat claustrophobic. However, it is an utterly extraordinary piece of technology, and (as with much of the machinery in a hospital) understanding how it works can be the key to feeling less nervous.

MRI stands for magnetic resonance imaging, and the machine uses magnets that are up to 3000 times stronger than a fridge magnet and up to 60,000 times stronger than the earth's magnetic field. Most of our body is made up of water molecules, within which are tiny particles called protons. These protons are very sensitive to magnetic fields, and when you lie under the powerful MRI scanner magnets, the protons in your body line up in the same direction, in the same way that a magnet pulls the needle of a compass. Short bursts of radio waves are then sent out by the scanner, knocking the protons out of alignment. When the radio waves are turned off, the protons realign, which also sends out radio signals. These signals from the millions of protons in your body are combined to create a detailed image on a screen. You need to keep extremely still so that the images are pin sharp, and the whole thing takes about half an hour. The water molecules in your body are being temporarily affected by the magnetism, but unlike CT or X-ray scans, there is no exposure to radiation, which makes it very safe. Sometimes a nurse will inject a dye into your veins beforehand to help them show up better on the images. The machine is constantly creating different magnetic fields and it makes an incredibly loud thumping, clanking noise as it shifts between them. The technicians will give you headphones to wear to cancel out the noise, and some hospitals will play you music.

Alan once went to sleep in the MRI scanner – possibly the

only person ever to do this, as even with the headphones on, the noise is still loud and disconcerting! This seemed like a good thing, as he was then completely still. Unfortunately, he woke up near the end of the scan and, because he didn't remember where he was, went into a panic and tried to sit up, which of course rendered the scan blurry and unusable! Because the magnets are so strong, you need to take off any metal items, such as belts or jewellery, before you go into the room; in fact, the staff usually ask you to change into a gown. In the early days, I always went into the MRI room with Alan to try and keep him calm.

One afternoon, as I come in, the technician notices that I haven't taken off my earrings, and I leave them just inside the door. After Alan's scan is over, I put them back on, and without thinking, step a little closer to the scanner. Suddenly I feel the most incredible force pulling me forward, which is actually rather frightening, like being under a magic spell. I quickly realise what it is and hastily step backwards, a little bit shaken. Afterwards, I read that heart monitors, drip stands, mops, buckets, vacuum cleaners and stretchers have all been accidentally pulled into MRI machines, so it seems that I had a lucky escape!

PET scan

Positron emission tomography (PET) scans are used to produce detailed three-dimensional images of the inside of your body. An advantage of a PET scan is that it can show how well certain parts of your body are working, rather than just showing what they look like. Before the scan, a substance called a radiotracer is injected into a vein in your arm or hand. The PET scanners work by detecting the radiation given off this radiotracer as it collects in different parts of your body. By analysing the areas where the radiotracer does and doesn't build up, it's possible to work out how well certain body functions are working and identify any abnormalities. In most PET scans, the radiotracer they use is similar to the glucose that your body produces naturally, so it treats it in a similar way. For example, a concentration of the radiotracer in the body's tissues can help identify cancerous cells because cancer cells use glucose at a much faster rate than normal cells. In a standard PET scan, the amount of radiation that you're exposed to is small and will be passed out of your body naturally within a few hours. A PET scan is often combined with a CT scan to produce even more detailed images and is known as a PET-CT scan.

Ultrasound scan

An ultrasound, sometimes called a sonogram, is a procedure that uses high-frequency sound waves to create an image of part of the inside of the body. A small device called an ultrasound probe is used, which gives off high-frequency sound waves. You can't hear these sound waves, but when they bounce off different parts of the body, they create 'echoes' that are picked up by the probe and turned into a moving image. This image is displayed on a monitor while the scan is carried out. Ultrasounds can be:

- external: where the probe is moved over your skin; this is used to look at unborn babies for example, or your heart, the organs in your abdomen or your muscles and joints

- internal: where the probe is gently passed into your vagina or rectum, allowing a doctor to look more closely at organs such as the prostate gland, ovaries or womb

- endoscopic: where the probe is attached to a long, thin, flexible tube (an endoscope) and passed through your mouth (usually) to examine areas such as your stomach.

X-ray

This is a quick and effective way of looking at your bones or teeth and can also be used to help detect a range of other issues. X-rays are a type of radiation and you can't see or feel them. A detector picks up the X-rays as they pass through you and turns them into an image. Dense parts of your body that X-rays find more difficult to pass through, such as bone, show up as clear white areas, and softer parts that the X-rays can pass through more easily, such as your heart and lungs, show up as darker areas.

The rise of the machines

The sheer amount of machinery available in the 21st-century hospital is pretty staggering. As well as scanners, some of the other vital bits of technology are:

- breathing machines or ventilators, which use complex computers to enable patients to breathe as much as possible for themselves with variable amounts of help from the machine

- defibrillators, which are devices that restore a normal heartbeat by sending an electric pulse or shock to the heart

- kidney machines, which can filter the blood and remove

waste products from a patient if their kidneys aren't working

- monitors, which among other things can measure a patient's heart rate, oxygen levels in the blood, urine output, blood pressure, temperature and all the fluids, food and drugs that go into them

- radiotherapy machines, which are used to carefully aim beams of radiation at cancer in the body

- plasma exchange machines, which are used for problems caused by abnormal antibodies or proteins in your blood, including some autoimmune disorders and some cancers. Blood is made up of red blood cells, white blood cells and platelets, all held in a liquid called plasma, which also contains the antibodies and proteins. The machine uses something called a blood cell separator, which separates and removes the plasma, taking with it the antibodies and proteins. It does this using centrifugal force, which means taking out your blood via a vein and then whizzing it round and round at a high speed in a contraption that looks and sounds a lot like a spin dryer! You can see the orangey yellow plasma pumping out into a bag. At the same time, clean fresh bottles (which look like dry sherry) of plasma made from donated blood are pumped back in, at the same time as the rest of your blood (including the red and white cells). Only a small amount of your blood passes through the machine at one time (about the same amount as a mug of coffee) but it's all happening at once, so it's very noisy! To 'clean' his blood of unwanted antibodies, Alan was hooked up to this machine all day, every day, for five days; and every day, 12 bottles of new plasma went in and 12 bottles of 'old' plasma came out. This extraordinary contraption was invented by American biochemist Edwin J. Cohn, who modified a machine used in Swedish dairies in the late 1800s for separating cream from milk!

Phones in hospitals

One of the most sophisticated machines inside a hospital will actually be the one that you have in your own pocket! The rules on how you can use it on the ward are changing fast, and different hospitals will have different regulations. The NHS recommends that every trust should have its own written policy, and you can ask to see this. Here are some general guidelines.

- You are allowed to record conversations with your doctor or nurse. The guidelines for hospitals produced by the Information Governance Alliance (IGA) say that 'the use of mobile devices by patients to capture details of or record their own consultations...is increasingly an accepted practice'. Staff must 'ensure that they continue to deliver appropriate care even where they are uncomfortable about this being recorded'.
- It is essential that you are sensitive to other people and any photos you take should definitely not include any other patients or visitors. The dignity and safety of all patients should be your primary concern.
- Studies have found high bacterial contamination, including MRSA, on mobile phones. To minimise

the risk, if you've been using your phone then you should wash your hands before you come into direct contact with a patient. And clean your phone frequently using antibacterial wipes.

- Signs will tell you where you cannot use your phone. Areas where using mobile phones may be forbidden or restricted include ICUs and special-care baby units.

- Interference from mobile phones can stop some medical equipment from working properly. Some of the machines this may affect includes dialysis machines, defibrillators and ventilators. If you're in any doubt – ask!

- A loud ringtone or an alarm on a mobile phone could be confused with the alarms on medical equipment. Probably best to keep it on silent.

- If you're not allowed to use your phone, make sure you switch it off. Don't just leave it on the silent or vibrate setting as that can still affect medical equipment.

- Charging your phone can be tricky – most of the plug sockets are in use! If you have a friend or relative in hospital, buying them a portable phone charger – and then taking that home to charge it up for them on a regular basis – would be a helpful thing to do.

- You must ensure that the use of your phone doesn't cause a nuisance to other people on the ward. If you want to listen to music or watch films, headphones are essential. If a patient is confined to bed, 'over-the-head' headphones are much better than small regular earphones as they don't get knocked out by pillows or blankets so easily. They would be a good present for someone in hospital.

- If you are recording or taking photos, things to consider are: the impact on a patient's right to privacy; any breach of confidentiality; any threat to safeguarding arrangements for children and vulnerable adults; any interruption to care provision; the creation of unacceptable working conditions for staff; undermining patient comfort and recuperation.

Chapter Seven

ALL HAIL THE HOSPITAL

A force for good

A HOSPITAL IS A TRULY extraordinary place, with a profound humanity at its heart. There have probably been 'hospitals' almost as long as there have been people, but their documented history goes back over 2500 years.

The diversity of a hospital strikes you every time you enter. There will always be someone both better and worse off than you. And as Christie Watson says in her wonderful book about nursing, *The Language of Kindness*, 'In the NHS the staff completely reflect the patients they serve, the nurses, doctors, porters, healthcare assistants, catering staff, cleaners and technicians come from all corners of the world – every background, race, culture and religion possible.'

Hospitals are purely a force for good; there is no malice, no meanness, no spite. The abiding principle of loving your neighbour that underpins pretty much all the major world religions is central to the way a hospital is run. Much of what happens in a hospital is undocumented, but these millions of invisible moments add up to millennia of compassion and care.

A very short hospital history

- In both Ancient Egypt and Greece, religion and medicine were inexorably linked. In Ancient Greece, temples dedicated to the healer-god Asclepius became centres of medical advice and healing, and in one, three large marble slabs from 350 BC are inscribed with the names, case histories and cures of about 70 patients.

- The earliest documentary evidence of institutions specifically dedicated to the care of the sick is in the *Mahavamsa*, an epic poem relating the history of Sri Lanka, written in the 6th century. There are still ruins of ancient hospitals in Sri Lanka.

- The Greek physician Hippocrates, often described as the 'father of Western scientific medicine' and credited with separating medicine from the supernatural and the divine, was born in 460 BC.

- Fa Xian, a Chinese Buddhist monk who travelled across India in around 400 AD, recorded that in cities there were 'houses for dispensing charity and medicine. All who are diseased, go to those houses, and are provided with every kind of help, and doctors examine their diseases.'

- The Romans constructed buildings called 'valetudinaria' for the care of sick gladiators and soldiers in around 100 BC, but it was not until Christianity became an accepted religion within the Roman

Empire that the expansion of hospitals for civilians really began.

- Galen of Pergamon (physician to Roman Emperor Marcus Aurelius) was born in 129 BC. He became the accepted medical authority in Western medicine for over a millennium.

- By the beginning of the 5th century, the hospital was ubiquitous in the Byzantine world. By the 12th century, Constantinople had established itself as a centre of medicine, with two well-organised hospitals and facilities that included systematic treatments and specialised wards for different diseases.

- The first hospitals in a Muslim country were built in the early 8th century to contain leprosy, but the first record of a hospital as a teaching centre was in Baghdad in the 900s. In 980, Avicenna, the Persian philosopher, physician and author of the *Canon of Medicine*, was born. The Islamic hospital was more elaborate than its Christian equivalent, with a wider range of functions, and was largely secular. It functioned as a centre of medical treatment, a place for patients to recover, an asylum for the insane and a home for the old and infirm.

- Medieval hospitals in Europe were usually within religious communities, with care provided by monks and nuns. An old French term for hospital is 'hôtel-Dieu', meaning 'hostel of God', and a hospital with this name in Paris, which was founded in 650, is thought to be the oldest hospital in the world that is still operating today.

- The Reformation brought about the secularisation of hospitals. In 1534, Henry VIII closed many of the larger hospitals along with the monasteries in England, and this meant that many had to be funded via charity. The important role that charity plays in medical care continues in Britain to this day.
- Following the French Revolution in 1789, the centre of Western medicine moved to Paris. The vast Parisian hospitals were huge – there were more hospital beds (20,000) in Paris in 1800 than there were in the whole of England. The access to such a huge number of clinical cases led doctors to make major advances in new diagnostic techniques.
- In 1847, Hungarian obstetrician Ignaz Semmelweis, working at a Vienna maternity hospital, instituted mandatory handwashing after hypothesising that medical students were infecting patients. This caused infection rates to drop dramatically.
- Florence Nightingale in the mid-1800s recognised the importance of hospital design in improving patients' health and recommended the layout of a long room, with a large window at one end for sunlight and fresh air, that is still the model for many hospital wards today. It was also her firm opinion that 'the greater part of nursing consists in preserving cleanliness'.
- During the 1860s, Louis Pasteur in France and

Robert Koch in Germany identified the germ origins of infectious diseases. In the same decade, surgeon Joseph Lister developed the use of antiseptic surgical methods, which heralded a revolution in surgical safety.

- From the late 19th century onwards, the services that hospitals could offer changed dramatically, due to scientific and technological innovations, such as the introduction of X-rays. Radium treatment for cancer was another important advance, as were the changes brought about by improved medical equipment, electric lighting and central heating.

- In 1928, Scottish scientist Alexander Fleming discovered the first antibiotic, penicillin, after noticing on a petri dish that the bacteria in close proximity to mould were dying.

- The NHS was founded by the minister of health, Aneurin Bevan, on 5 July 1948. It had at its heart three core principles: that it meets the needs of everyone; that it be free at the point of delivery; and that it be based on clinical need, not ability.

What I've learnt about the UK healthcare system

I have learnt that you are ultimately in charge of your own welfare. Paying your taxes or living in the UK does not mean you can be absolved of all responsibility for your own wellbeing. The NHS may be there for you 'from cradle to grave', but it is a huge, sprawling mass of an organisation, and the person who should know most about your health is not your GP or consultant, it is you. An online system called Patients Know Best (sometimes referred to as PKB or CIE: the Care Information Exchange) has been created in partnership with the NHS and is designed to bring together data from health and social care providers and the patient's own information into one secure personal health record. If you are offered this option, I would recommend that you take it. When the system was introduced in West Birmingham, for example, up to 98% of patients said PKB 'enhanced the relationship with their clinical team'. And taking control will not just make you healthier, it will make you happier too.

I have learnt that nurses and doctors are not angels or gods, and to describe them as such is a bad idea. First, using saintly and sacred language about the NHS allows us to believe that its employees don't need proper materialistic things, like a salary and social life. And second, the 'they're all wonderful, altruistic guardians of the galaxy' view removes the possibility that some doctors and nurses are better at their jobs than others. There are great doctors, and there are OK doctors. There are good nurses, there are fairly good nurses and there are just a little bit rubbish nurses. And that's alright because they are all humans, just like the rest of us, and it's their job, not their calling.

I have learnt that you will need to 'join the dots'. The NHS will not do this for you. Most people have already taken charge of the health of their own nails, hair, teeth, eyes and ears. Some people extend that list to monitor their overall fitness and consider how well their digestive systems and reproductive organs are working. I would suggest we all need to think about our hearts, our lungs, our joints, our backs and our mental health. Most self-care doesn't require a doctor and is about prevention rather than cure.

I have learnt that while charities are extremely good at assimilating the stories and experiences of patients to make their information and support better, the NHS is not. As David Gilbert says in his thought-provoking book *The Patient Revolution*, 'decision-making is being made by stealth and in secret, partly because of fear about grown-up conversations'. All the hospitals Alan has been in have sent me endless 'tick-box' questionnaires about his care, but there is absolutely no feedback or indication that anyone who matters is looking at them. And, as Gilbert points out, 'patients are not permitted to eyeball the data or bring their own interpretation to it, let alone be partners in decisions about what to do'. He hopes that the 'wisdom gained through suffering' could lead to an 'enriched expertise in order to help others', and that is my hope too, but I see little sign of it.

I have learnt that even if you have a brilliant consultant who meets with you regularly and talks to you as if you are an intelligent equal, you will still never find out what is happening to all the medical information the hospital have assimilated about your case. Time and again, we were told how unusual Alan's condition was, how new all the science was and how few cases like his there were. But there is no system to tell you where all this knowledge goes. Were his notes discussed at academic conferences? Were the many medical students who met him now using his case to help diagnose other patients? Were doctors learning valuable lessons from the five months he was under their care? Was his experience adding to the sum of medical knowledge? It would have made a huge difference to us to feel we were part of the solution rather than just part of the problem.

I have learnt that most hospitals are incredibly confusing to find your way around. The genius of Google was realising that when you are on a quest for help, what you want to see is a clean white page. A well-designed office building or hotel is the same – all unnecessary signage has been removed to create a calm welcoming space. And this is exactly the vibe you want in a hospital, but every single one I've ever been in is totally baffling and full of confusing clutter. If I were in charge, I would remove all the notice boards, all the leaflets, all the maps, all the passive-aggressive notes about not being rude to staff, all the taxi info, all the long words for different clinics. Anyone walking into a hospital is ill, anxious, exhausted or in a hurry and possibly all of the above. What we want to see are clean white walls and just one huge sign saying something like 'Welcome to this hospital. We hope we can help you.' There should maybe be three more big signs, for A&E, Outpatients and Other Departments, with more information as you get further in. And best of all, you could have a couple of staff on hand to help people and direct them to where they need to go.

Not all hospitals are as bad. Here's a description of the Queen Elizabeth Hospital in Birmingham, from Jonathan Coe's novel *Middle England*: 'Inside, the enormous atrium, with its glass ceiling, induced a sense of calm and admiration, and even gentle optimism, so that for once the experience of entering a hospital did not result in an immediate lowering of the spirits. It was such a pleasant space that Sophie could imagine coming here just to visit the café, maybe to read a book and do some work.' Exactly. Please can more of them be like this?

Poem for a Hospital Wall, Diana Hendry

Love has been loitering
down this corridor
has been seen
chatting up out-patients

spinning the wheels of wheelchairs
fluttering the pulse of the night nurse
appearing, disguised, as a bunch of grapes and a smile
hiding in dreams
handing out wings in orthopedics
adding a wee drappie
aphrodisiaccy
to every prescription.
No heart is ever by-passed by Love.
Love has been loitering down this corridor
It's highly infectious
mind how you go. If you smile
you might catch it.

This poem appears by kind permission of the author. It was originally painted onto a corridor wall of Dumfries and Galloway Royal Infirmary, when Diana was Writer-in-Residence there, and is published in *Borderers*, Peterloo Poets.

Chapter Eight

IT'S A FAMILY AFFAIR

Talking and Listening to Children, Siblings and Parents

Spreading the word

THE MORNING AFTER ALAN'S first seizure, I am sitting up in bed at my parents' house, with my phone, next to a gently snoring Alan. The first thing I need to do is tell Lucy and Simon what has happened. The second thing I need to do is tell his sister, Ginny. And thus begins an ongoing process of disseminating information, which anyone who is looking after someone who is seriously ill will recognise. You love your family and want to keep them in the loop, but keeping everyone updated can be hugely time-consuming. There are ways you can make this easier...

Set up a WhatsApp group for close family, specifically for news about the illness. After a few weeks of writing masses of different text messages and emails, I created a new group that comprised me, all five of Alan's children and Ginny. Lucy was in Manchester, Simon in north London, Izzy in Cambridge,

Madeleine in Warwick and Ginny in Surrey; the only person I spoke to on a daily basis was Sam.

Some days I had very bad news to relay, some days it was more encouraging, but putting it all in one place meant that everyone could see it at the same time, digest it and, if necessary, refer to it later. Complex medical information can take a while to assimilate, and it can be far easier to take in facts if they are written down. This actually brought a major benefit to me, in that every time the doctors gave me some medical information, I had to summarise it to put on the group chat, which often clarified the situation in my own mind. The group made it easy to offer each other support and no one was worried about asking silly questions as, inevitably, someone else was thinking the same thing.

If you are the relative of someone who is ill but not the 'primary carer', offering to be the conduit to spread the information a bit further round the family is a very useful thing to do. My sister Alice took on this role, without my asking her, and it was enormously welcome. It meant that I could tell her things either on the phone or by text and then she relayed it outward to our large family. Trauma can mean your brain is struggling to process information, and you are unlikely to be in the mood to explain complicated things to distant relatives. If you plan on taking on this role, I recommend saying something like 'You have so much on your mind at the moment, shall I let everyone else in the family know what's happening?' People can sometimes feel almost embarrassed by medical things, so they may say something like 'Oh no, I'll give them a call when I've got a bit more information', but I would advise being quite firm and saying 'I won't give too many details if you don't want me to, but I think it will be better if everyone knows, and you don't need the hassle.' It's a huge relief when someone takes charge in this way, and there is usually nothing whatsoever to be gained from being secretive.

On the other hand, if you are the member of the family who finds out about the situation a bit later than you would have liked, please don't make anyone feel guilty about this! I received a few letters that were very kind but which I felt had a slightly accusatory tone, implying that I should have let them know about Alan's illness sooner. It genuinely doesn't mean that you are less important or less valued in the family if you find out later than other people. It is almost impossible to tell everyone everything, and when a family are in a state of shock, things sometimes get done in the wrong order or not done at all.

What is wonderful is when members of your family get in touch with messages of support, even when you haven't been directly in touch with them. I am lucky enough to have a very large family, and I cannot tell you how much it meant during a long day to get a text saying 'thinking of you' or to come home to find a card or a letter and sometimes a small present! Scottish tablet, Yorkshire fudge, Welsh cakes and many, many cards arrived from relations far and wide, and they made a big difference on horrible days. Small thoughtful gestures can be a big help, and the really good thing about an encouraging message is that you can reread it whenever you feel low.

Looking after each other

Lucy and Craig arrive for a visit, and as soon as I open the door, Craig gives me an absolutely massive bear hug. I think it might actually be the best hug I've ever had; its strength feels as if it is seeping into my very bones. One thing that Alan's illness has given to our family, I think, is that it has made us all better at caring for each other. We come to see that the pattern of who looks after whom isn't set in stone, and there will be times when we need support and times when we can give support.

As soon as Al goes into hospital, my parents, who are in their late seventies and might reasonably expect their daughter to be helping them, spring into action. My brilliant dad is a superman of support, regularly making the 200-mile round trip in his van to come and repair the myriad of things that go wrong in the house, as well as helping Sam with maths and science homework and cheering us both up. My wonderful mum often comes too and keeps us supplied with cakes, casseroles and other delicious homemade treats. Sometimes I look after my children and sometimes they look after me, just as is happening with my own parents. What has happened to Alan has undoubtably changed the dynamic of many of our family relationships, and I hope it has made them stronger.

Children and hospitals

When I started writing this book, my first discovery was that there are lots of picture books written to prepare children for a stay in hospital but nothing for adults. My second realisation was that although there are books for children who are going to be a patient, there is not much for those going into hospital as visitors. If you want a novel that vividly describes the hospital experience for children (and adults) and is an emotional but brilliantly uplifting read, I recommend Michael Morpurgo's *Cool!*

The power of youth

I am sitting in the hospital café feeling very low. Alan isn't making much progress, and I feel as if I don't know where things are going or where we'll end up. I can't think beyond the illness, the here and now, the endless grimness of it all.

Suddenly I hear two little voices shouting, 'Granny! Granny!' Nancy and Esther, my small granddaughters, bowl through the café and hug me. I almost can't believe they are here; their vibrant chirpiness, their noisiness, their littleness, their sheer healthiness all seem completely alien in this world of sadness and bad news. Maddy, my stepdaughter-in-law, smiles apologetically, 'Sorry, Simon's up visiting Al and it just didn't work with the girls there too.' I am so overjoyed to see them that I can hardly speak. 'Perfect,' I say. 'This café has really nice brownies, let's have some tea and cakes.'

The girls are very pleased: this afternoon has taken a definite turn for the better. They chat and chat about their lives and, listening to them, I can almost physically feel the cloak of misery lifting off my shoulders. They are so utterly unconcerned about their surroundings, the fact that on every other table there are people looking stressed; all they can see is the unexpected joy of chocolate cake and being the centre of attention for a while. After a while, Simon comes down from the ward, his face weary with worry about his dad. 'I hope they haven't been too much,' he says. 'They've been absolutely brilliant,' I say. I feel as if they've pulled me out of a swamp, and it's made a huge difference having them there. Today, their visit might not have benefitted Alan, but it certainly has me.

Bringing young children into a hospital environment can be challenging: they get bored and fractious easily and there is usually not much space to move around. But the power they hold to lift everyone's spirits really cannot be underestimated. Alan's first meeting with our new grandson, George, takes place in hospital, and in the photograph we took to mark the occasion, you can see him, slightly bemused but still looking like the confident and jolly little lad he is, sitting on Alan's lap as he lies in bed. Unseen beneath the bedcovers is the tangle of tubes connected to Alan, ready for the plasma exchange.

There is a great deal of research showing what a positive effect bringing primary school children into care homes can have. Studies claim that this type of interaction, often referred to as 'intergenerational care', can decrease older people's loneliness, delay mental decline, lower blood pressure and even reduce the risk of disease or death.

Lesley Carter, from the charity Age UK, said, 'I have seen it so often, when a child touches the hand of somebody who is perhaps very withdrawn, and not really speaking, and all of a sudden that person is alive. It's really humbling.' Other carers talk about how toddlers make patients 'light up' and boost their feeling of 'self-worth'. My sister Alice works with a project in Cornwall, where school children visit homes to make music with people living with dementia and Alzheimer's, and has seen first-hand how immensely rewarding an experience it can be, for both sides.

If you are old or ill, being with small children brings you back into the world, connecting you immediately to the present, as well as the future. Being isolated and, even worse, feeling incarcerated are some of the very worst things for anyone's mental health. Ensuring that children have people in their lives who are elderly, and maybe unwell, helps normalise both age and ill health. And undoubtably, it will help them to grow into more empathetic, caring human beings.

Surveys (2018) have shown that children under eight are much less likely to hypothesise about the outcome of an illness than older children and tend to be more interested in the practical rather than the emotional issues. They will take their cues from the adults around them, so if you're not scared and sad, there's a good chance that they won't be either.

Tips for talking to young children

- Talk about the practicalities. Little children are usually fascinated by machines and tubes and are much less fazed by bodily functions than adults. Explain everything.
- Treat it as a learning experience. Children love to find out new things.
- Sort out misunderstandings early. Ask them questions after talking to or visiting a patient, and gently correct them if they have got the wrong end of the stick.
- Prepare to have more than one conversation about the illness.
- Don't make any one discussion longer than about ten minutes.
- Look for their cues. Be ready to answer questions when they have them, even if they come out of the blue or at an inconvenient time. And if they suddenly stop wanting to talk about it, that is their way of needing time to process what you've said; it doesn't mean they are bored. Be led by them.
- Give them information in advance about what to

> expect, especially when visiting a new environment. Focus on how things will look.
> - Make sure they understand that this is nothing whatsoever to do with anything they've done or said.

Older children

Helping teenagers to process their feelings about illness is very difficult. From speaking to friends who have been in a similar situation, and reading advice from child psychologists, it is clear that there are many different ways of coping – and not coping. Like some adults, some teenagers will want to compartmentalise the entire experience, to put the illness 'in a box' and get on with their lives while trying not to think about it. Others may be on an endless quest for information, feeling that forewarned is forearmed. Some may internalise it and insist they don't want to talk, only to break down months later. Some may become much more erratic and emotional, others quieter and more studious. Most will utilise a combination of these strategies. And, less often but sometimes, a child can find the unpredictable nature of illness just too hard to cope with and may develop a mental health issue, such as an eating disorder, as a way of regaining some control over a frightening situation.

As a parent, you want to make everything alright for your children, and I found it very hard to accept that I was not necessarily going to be able to 'solve' this problem. The emotional fallout from serious illness can take a long time to deal with and there is no 'one size fits all' answer. However, I do think it is vital to acknowledge what's happening, even if you feel you are being rebuffed, and I know my children found it most upsetting when other adults in the family didn't mention Alan at all. People's reasons for not mentioning illness are kind ones, but in my experience, saying something is better than saying nothing.

Thoughts on talking to teenagers

- There isn't necessarily a 'right time' to talk. It's often hard to find enough time or the ideal moment to discuss things in depth. In my experience, it's better to fumble through and get it wrong than let things build up. You can have several tries at explaining something.
- If you don't have an answer to their question, say you don't know. One of the hardest lessons to learn about illness is that there aren't always answers.
- Have a sense of certainty about what you are doing. Even if the plan is just 'we are going to take each day as it comes', make sure you convey this. Young people do not want to feel cut adrift, and it is important to show them that the parental relationship is still in place.
- As with other issues, a car journey is a good time and place to talk to a teenager, as you are in close proximity but not looking at each other. And they can't walk away.
- Try to strike a balance within your family between positivity and realism. You can be truthful about the

seriousness of the situation but also be constructive about how you and they will cope with it.

- It is OK for your child to see that you are upset and worried, and this may help them express their own feelings. Make sure that you tell them you are sad because of the illness and not because of anything they've done.
- Be aware that the other things children have in their lives, such as other relationships or exams, are still going on. These may be providing a welcome distraction, but they may also be causing additional worry.
- Emotions in your household will be running high. This heightened tension may well result in arguments about seemingly unconnected things. This is OK.
- Give them reliable sources of information to refer to; the hospital will usually have leaflets, or you can buy a book. Do not let them get all their information about the illness from the internet, which is very likely to be wrong.
- Ask another member of your family to talk to them and ask how they are feeling. Do this even if your children appear to be fine, as it is often hard for them to tell their parents what they are worried about.
- If your teenager is at a point where they are ready to spread their wings and the illness disrupts this, try to make them feel that these sacrifices are acknowledged and appreciated.
- If you have more than one child, they will each

have different emotional and physical capabilities. Don't treat them the same way or compare them to each other.
- Children may not want to tell their friends. This is fine. It may help them keep some normality in their lives, and it must be their decision.
- You may not be equipped to help your teenager on your own, and you should not feel as if you have failed if you need to seek professional help. Your GP is probably the best place to start.
- Everyone's relationship to the ill person will be different. So, remember that each member of the family will have their own unique sense of loss.

Allowing children to be brave

It's Friday morning and half term, so Sam is with me. As we arrive, Dr Lander greets me, fizzing with enthusiasm. We have rapidly begun to notice that there are various 'types' of doctor. Dr Lander is one of those whose name you feel is frequently prefixed by 'that nice young'. He is good looking, with glasses and a puppy-ish eagerness, and in short is the sort of doctor that everyone imagines they want. He has already rung me the evening before to say that he has good news, and as soon as we arrive, he ushers me into his office. I look at Sam. 'Will you be OK seeing Dad without me? I won't be very long.' He nods, a nurse smiles at me reassuringly; the staff on the ward all know him by now.

I go into a small office, which I realise much later on is

extremely unusual – most medical conversations, even the most painful or private, take place on the ward, in a corridor or in the hallway next to the lifts. Dr Lander is telling me that he has got the approval of the faceless and nameless powers that be to give Alan a powerful drug called Rituximab, which should zap the rogue antibodies that are in his blood and will hopefully return him to 'normal'. In order to establish that Alan is a sensible candidate for this medicine, he has Googled him and, there on his computer screen, is Al's company website. This confirms that he is indeed the MD of a successful business, providing sales and marketing services to publishers, and was until very recently what Dr Lander describes as 'a high-functioning executive'. I am, in fact, the creator of this website, and although I don't tell Dr Lander this, I feel no small degree of satisfaction that what's on the screen is good enough to prove that Alan is worthy of the special drug. At the same time though, I wonder what happens to those who aren't deemed to be 'an ideal candidate for treatment'. Already, we seem to be in some dystopian version of *Catch-22*, where in order to prove that you have gone mad, you have to be able to show that you weren't mad already. And if you don't have a non-mad person at your side to tell doctors this, how would they know?

At that moment, a nurse pokes her head round the door. 'Are you nearly done? I think your son could do with some assistance.' Dr Lander looks a bit annoyed at having been interrupted. 'Umm, I'll just check he's OK,' I say.

Out on the ward, things are not going well. Alan has put on Sam's green puffer jacket (although it is far too small for him) over his hospital gown and is carrying my red, patent leather handbag on one arm. He is walking round and round in circles, with an almost comedically cross look on his face. I am immediately reminded of a *Tintin* book, and a page where a man has been injected with a poison that makes him go instantly and irreversibly mad. I look at Sam and I know that he is frightened. I'm frightened too. The nurse can't persuade Alan to go back to bed, and he looks disturbingly bizarre. 'Can you manage for a moment? I just need a bit longer with Dr Lander.' 'Ye-e-ss, I think so.' Hospitals are the steepest of learning curves, and I see my 13-year-old boy growing up before my eyes. I see that he is scared – but I also see that he is coping. In amongst the intense worry and all the questions that are whirring around in my head to ask Dr Lander, I feel extraordinarily and emotionally proud of him. 'I won't be long. You're doing great.'

Building family resilience

It is July, and I am with Madeleine at a conference organised by the Encephalitis Society at The Royal Society of Medicine, entitled *Encephalitis: My Brain and Me*. It is incredibly informative and incredibly emotional. There are around a hundred people in the lecture hall. Some are family members like us, but many have had encephalitis themselves and it seems extraordinary to think that Alan would ever be well enough to come to something like this. And yet just being in a room with people who have come through it gives us hope. A young woman speaks movingly about her experience, and we feel humbled by her bravery and pragmatism; she is very far from recovered but she is determined to live as full a life as she can.

The medical science talks are absorbing too; there is a Power-Point screen showing a visual representation of the 'rogue' GABA B antibodies in Alan's bloodstream, and the science is so new that this is the first time we have actually seen it properly written down, properly explained. I take a photo to put on our WhatsApp chat. Then comes the talk we are really looking forward to, 'Building Family Resilience Following Encephalitis' by Dr Audrey Daisley. This is a clinical neuropsychologist who has worked with children after someone in the family has had encephalitis.

She talks at length about the effect on all the families, the trauma and the shock. But the most striking thing she tells us is that the current therapeutic research is focusing on a small number of families who have come through the experience in the best shape. She quotes a researcher called Walsh (2006) who said that the families who coped best were those who were 'struggling well, effectively working through and learning from adversity... and integrating the experience into the fabric of individual and shared lives'. When she puts the screen up showing the things that such families are doing, Mads and I read it and then turn to each other, eyes full of tears. 'Mum, that's us. You're doing that.' 'We're all doing that,' I reply. We both choke up, clasping hands.

It is such an affirmation to see that, although we're still wading through the mire of Alan's illness, we seem to be on the right track. There's lots more good advice on the screen and it feels like the first time someone has acknowledged scientifically that having a positive outlook can genuinely give patients and their families a better outcome.

By now, Alan has moved from hospital to a Brain Injury Rehabilitation Centre, and we're all coming to terms with the fact that the doctors, the science and the medicine cannot completely cure Alan and he will never be back to 'normal'. But going to the conference shows Madeleine and me that we are not the only ones on this journey. And that evening when we pass on all the information to Sam, Izzy, Simon and Lucy, it makes us all proud of the way we've coped so far and proud of our support for one another.

Dr Daisley's strategies

These ideas are for families of patients with brain injuries, but I think that most of them would be equally useful for any family learning to live with a serious illness. A phrase she used that I especially liked was not to try and 'bounce back' but instead to 'bounce forward'.

The tactic adopted by traditional rehabilitation can tend to focus on problems to be 'fixed' by the professionals, asking families to provide accounts of 'what's gone wrong'. Typically, this puts the emphasis on failure and not on success. Dr Daisley and her team are pioneering a different approach.[1]

Building a resilient family

- A family that can withstand and rebound from life challenges will emerge strengthened and more resourceful.
- Place an emphasis on collaboration, openness and shared goals.
- Look for family strengths and solutions, not problems.
- The whole family should feel heard and have the chance to tell their story.

1   Reproduced with kind permission from Audrey Daisley.

- It can help to look at previous stories of adversity and how it was managed.
- Put an emphasis on 'good-enough' coping.
- Focus on normalising ambivalence and negative feelings.
- The family need to develop ways to accept and live with uncertainty.
- It is possible to rethink ideas of who does what within the family.
- Discourage pre-injury comparison and use one week after the illness began as a marker for progress, not the patient's pre-injury self.
- Use humour.
- Resilient families tend to have an optimistic bias, with an awareness of the 'grim reality' but confidence that they can overcome problems and that things will improve.
- Reframing the illness as a shared family challenge that has meaning or purpose can contribute to the family's growth, strength and closeness.

Making happy memories

A couple of years later, I get around to printing out photos from my phone of all the other things we've done in 2017 as well as visiting Alan, and I put them into an album. There's the day trip Madeleine, Sam and I had to Brighton, the day I went to Cambridge with Mads to visit Izzy and we swam in the Cam, visits from relations, sunny days in the garden, family parties, my friend Jane's wedding. There's Izzy's graduation, the children's birthdays, the week the kids and I had in Mallorca. It's an odd feeling to see so many smiling, happy pictures, when overall, the year has been such a dreadful one. But the pictures remind us all that there were lots and lots of cheery times in between the stress and the worry. I stick them in chronologically, interspersed with photos of us and Alan in hospital, and in fact, most of these have smiling faces in too. Of course, we all have our own recollections from 2017, of the very worst times. But it feels important to keep a physical record of the good days, the happy memories.

When kids become carers

Towards the end of the year, I am standing in the kitchen with a good friend and we're talking about how we will cope when Alan leaves the rehab centre. I'm telling her that I worry about how much I've leant on Sam and how much more he'll have to do when Al is back at home. The main issue is going to be that Alan can't be left alone or he gets anxious or confused, or wanders. The staff in the Brain Rehab Centre are not at all sure that we will be able to manage. I can see that when it is just Sam and me, it is going to mean that Sam has to look after his dad sometimes, otherwise I am never going to be able to leave the house. My friend turns to me, her face creased with concern. 'Oh Catherine,' she says. 'You can't turn Sam into a carer, it isn't fair on him.' I love my friend dearly, but right at that moment, I feel like strangling her.

For Sam, the effects are seismic. He goes, almost overnight, from being a child with a fully active 'normal' dad to a child with a dad who will need full-time care for the rest of his life. Alan has been a father who is fun, who is busy, who works long hours, but is social, chatty, active; who takes Sam on camping trips, drives him to five-a-side and Sunday league football matches, where he stands on the touchline cheering with the other dads. Now he does none of those things. He is tired, often talks nonsense, is sometimes withdrawn and is often, in his own words, 'bewildered' by his own change in circumstances. So far, he still hasn't come to terms with the fact that Sam is now taking care of him, rather than the other way around; something that Sam himself had to adapt to almost instantly.

In 2018, a BBC News report asked nearly a thousand 11–15-year-olds to fill in a survey and found that more than a fifth (22%) of them provided some care for a family member with an illness or disability. That could potentially mean that there are as many as 800,000 young carers in England, with six young carers in every secondary school classroom. Reading this makes me appreciate that Sam is not alone; there are many other children out there helping their disabled parents or siblings. As I realised with my friend that day, there is often no practical alternative to this situation.

Tips for kids who are carers

- Your child is being asked to grow up faster than they should. Try to balance their extra responsibilities by giving them some extra leeway on other things. Their early maturity should bring them some benefits as well as losses.

- But don't abandon all rules completely! When a child's world tips off kilter, the need for adults to behave consistently and with authority is vital.
- Don't worry that kids don't want their friends to know that they have to look after their parent. This embarrassment is normal.
- Make sure they have something fun to do on their downtime. I'd always been pretty strict about video and computer games (i.e., no, you're not having them), but when a relative offered a free PlayStation 3, I jumped at it.
- Tell teachers at school what the situation is. In my experience, kids absolutely hate people knowing things like this, but it is vital that you keep other adults in the loop.
- Instil in your child a sense that what they are doing is valued and important. Ensure they know that they should be extremely proud of themselves and that you are proud of them.

Chapter Nine

YOU'VE GOT A FRIEND IN ME

Assembling an Army

Read all about it – breaking news

ONE OF THE BEST things I ever did during the early days was to send a group email to about 25 of my friends and neighbours. This perhaps seems rather odd, as if I'm in the habit of sending 'round-robin' Christmas letters, which I'm not. But I realised almost straight away that I was going to be bumping into people in the street, on the bus or at the shops, and it was going to be absolutely awful to have to tell the whole story again and again. I also knew I wasn't going to have the time and energy to help with neighbourhood, church or school stuff for a while, and rather selfishly, I wanted to make sure people knew why.

So, I started 'Dear friends, please excuse the mass email...' and just gave everyone the facts. The huge advantage of this was that messages of support immediately came pouring back into my inbox. If you don't fancy sending an email, maybe consider telling the most talkative person in the street and asking them to actively spread the news that someone in your family is seriously ill. I think people would much rather know what's happening than accidentally say something insensitive out of ignorance. Lots of people told me that they were very pleased to know that I was not trying to battle on in silence, and it also meant that I had a little army of supporters who offered to help me, which proved immensely useful.

The good neighbours

I think there is a big old myth that everyone else's neighbours are better than yours. In fact, most of us probably live in a road where we only know a few people by name and a few more people to nod to. But I think that, given the chance, most people are only too ready to extend the hand of friendship. After sending the email about Alan's illness, word spread, and before long, complete strangers were stopping me in the street to ask, 'How's your husband?' And this is in a city often slated as unfriendly. Our knights in shining armour weren't confined to the neighbours we knew best, and it certainly taught me something about making assumptions. Lots dropped round food, and all sorts of yummy treats arrived, from home baking to an entire roast dinner! Some brought round books to take to Alan; one offered to help with any car fixing issues I might have, which was incredibly thought-ful; one came to my rescue in the middle of the night when a pipe burst! Many just always went out of their way to ask how I was and say how well they thought I was doing, which was an enormous boost. You never get the chance to say how much you appreciate these things at the time – but to all my lovely friends and neighbours, you know who you are – THANK YOU!

Alan's many friends in the book industry also provided much support and love – particularly his own team of reps. Alan's beloved company car (a Seat Alhambra) was reallocated to the Northern Account Manager, Dave, and to help Alan come to terms with the concept that he was no longer driving it, I asked Dave if he could WhatsApp me pictures of him and the car in various UK locations. Dave took to this task with gusto, and the 'Seat Selfies', as we dubbed them, always made us smile.

So, how should you respond when a friend tells you that they are, or someone in their family is, seriously ill? This is not a 'one size fits all' issue, but there are certainly pitfalls to avoid. I would say that the dangers lie in being too negative, but also, oddly, too positive.

The dangers of being too positive

'Dear Catherine, we are thinking of you and your family. What an awful shock for you all. Please do let us know if there is anything we can do at all. Somehow, I feel in my bones that Alan will be OK.'

'Hi Catherine, just wanted you to know that I heard someone talking on the radio this morning about encephalitis, and they were really ill, but they made a complete recovery. Alan is such a strong person; I just know he will pull through this.'

Two texts sent shortly after Alan became ill. Well meaning and kind, yes. Remotely helpful, no. It is certainly true that it is always better to say something than say nothing; and something good rather than bad also seems like a good idea. But beware a tone that is too upbeat; you cannot possibly know how any illness will turn out, and it can be extremely hurtful to make predictions.

I am very aware that with my propensity for jolly optimism, I will almost certainly have put my foot in it big time in the past. Hopefully, I have learnt from my blunders and I now strongly believe that the key to talking to someone who is seriously ill is to not, on any account, speculate about the future. Focus on the present. Much better to say 'You are doing so well. I can't imagine how difficult it is, but from where I am standing, you are coping brilliantly.' I think this applies whether you are talking to the patient or the carer. I probably tell Alan at least twice a day how well he is doing, and to be honest, the most helpful thing for me is when someone else tells me how well *I'm* doing!

Five things to say to a friend who is ill

- I don't really know what to say, but I am very sorry to hear your news.
- Please let me know what I can do to help. I was thinking of... [insert something that you genuinely can do].
- We are all thinking of you. Call any time – I mean that.
- Whatever happens, know that we are there for you.
- Here is [insert small gift] for you.

Five things *not* to say to a friend who is ill

- You are such a lucky person, so I'm sure you will be OK.
- Whatever happens, it is God's will.
- I will pop round later to see if there is anything I can do.
- I heard someone talking about this, and apparently there are some fantastic new drugs available.
- It's amazing what doctors can do nowadays.

The dangers of being too negative

'Hi Catherine, I am so, so sorry. To be honest I can't really talk about it, as I just keep bursting into tears when I think about what you are going through.'

'Oh hi, I hear your dad's really ill? It must be so awful, can you tell me a bit more about it, I don't really know anything about encephalitis? It sounds really scary, is it like he's just gone mad?'

I'm afraid that you will probably have friends – and even members of your family – who appear to take an almost ghoulish interest in your illness, and the more serious it is, the more sympathetic they become. Both of the above remarks are genuine, the latter one made to my daughter by another mother whom she'd never met before, during what should have been a fun evening. If someone looks wobbly and upset and you're a close friend, a hug or an arm round a shoulder can work wonders. But if they seem to be putting a brave face on it, it's your role to support them with that. Another gaffe to avoid is posting sad comments on your friend's social media accounts when they haven't mentioned the illness online.

I found a sympathetic smile, or a quick clasp of a shoulder, to be so much more helpful than public weeping and wailing. Remember, someone else's ill health is not an opportunity to virtue signal your own empathy. It is also not an opportunity to find out the gory details – if that's your thing, the internet is ready and waiting.

Reach out

There are lots of ways to let people know that you're thinking of them. The list below contains all things that friends did that were very much appreciated. You often don't get the chance to thank people properly for reaching out when times are tough, but be assured that showing someone that you're thinking of them provides a huge boost on difficult days.

The important thing is not to be offended if an offer of help is turned down or if you don't get a thank you.

Staying in touch

- Suggest a walk. It is best to make this fairly immediate; otherwise it won't happen. So, you could say something like 'I'm off for a walk along the river, do

> you fancy coming? I'm quite flexible on timings, so any time today would be OK if right now is tricky?'
> - Ask if they want to go to a gallery with you.
> - Or to see a film.
> - Send a silly text or email a joke.
> - Send a postcard if you are away somewhere.

Write a letter

It is difficult to find the right card to send to someone who is ill, especially if you don't know exactly how ill they are. The shops have a huge variety of get-well soon cards from the sorrowfully sympathetic, to the crudely comic, and if you can't find one that you're certain is just right, a card without a printed message is much the better option. And even better than a get-well-soon card might be writing a short letter. People don't do this much these days, but a chatty letter can be a powerful tonic. You might worry that you haven't got anything to say, but just wittering on about what you have been doing – however ordinary – is incredibly soothing to read, and visualising a life away from the world of illness is very therapeutic.

If you are writing to someone in hospital, put their full name on the envelope and then 'patient' in brackets, the ward name and the full address of the hospital, including the postcode. If you are the carer for a patient, it's a really good idea to bring a folder into hospital so that the patient can keep all their cards and letters in one place. Things go missing in hospital a lot, and it's easy for letters to get swept up with old newspapers and so on by the cleaners.

You don't bring me flowers

Since around 1996, most NHS hospitals haven't permitted visitors to bring in flowers. There are various reasons for this. The most quoted is that of the threat from bacteria in the water in the vase as the flowers decay, but although a 1973 study had found high counts of bacteria in flower water, subsequent research found that 'there was no evidence that flower water has ever caused hospital acquired infection'.

However, there are plenty of other practical reasons for not allowing vases of flowers, such as: the bedside curtains knocking over vases, resulting in broken glass on the floor; staff not having time to change the water; spilt water causing falls; pollen causing hay fever. The *Daily Mail* harrumphed in a 2009 article that 'hospitals are wrong to ban flowers as a health threat' and insisted that 'hospitals that ban flowers in an attempt to stop infections spreading are actually slowing patients' recovery'. Nevertheless, unless you are in a private hospital, it is unlikely that flowers will be welcome on the ward.

But that doesn't mean that you can't give flowers to the family of the person who is in hospital, and I would highly recommend that you do!

Perfect presents for hospital patients

- Fruit. Grapes are the traditional choice – but whatever you choose, please make it something that a patient will want to eat! Hard oranges or soft apples will sit around for ages looking sad and will then be thrown away by the nurse. When I was in hospital following a caesarean to have Izzy, my mum and dad brought in some raspberries from their garden, and they were the most delicious things I'd ever tasted. Satsumas are also good because the citrusy smell is so invigorating. Which brings me on to...

- Perfume. A spritz of something uplifting like rosewater or lavender can be a really good way to transport yourself away from the clinical ward environment.

- Photographs. These are a lovely thing to bring someone, as they can evoke happier times. A study in *Nature* magazine (2015) showed that recalling positive memories could reverse depression, and photographs are a great way of summoning up those good times. When Alan was in his own room, we put lots of pictures of friends and family up on the wall. We were doing this primarily to try and improve his memory, but it would be a good thing to do for any patient, as it made the surroundings so much nicer. Old family photo albums can also be a great thing to lend to someone in bed.

- Hand cream. Hospitals will have bottles of hand

gel all over the place, but something that smells gorgeous and is moisturising is a welcome gift.

- A tempting soft drink. Patients often don't drink enough water and a bottle of flavoured squash or cordial can really help with that. Make it something extra appealing and a bit luxurious, rather than own-brand orange; it's good to feel spoilt when you are ill!
- A book is invaluable, and a magazine is excellent too.
- Biscuits. Try to make these as delicious as you can possibly bake or afford; the hospital will give patients biscuits with their teas and coffee, but they are pretty unexciting!
- Enabling someone in hospital to listen to music is a real boon. Anyone under the age of 50 will certainly be able to listen to music on their phone, but someone older possibly won't. When my dad went into hospital, I gave him a portable CD player with some classical music CDs, which shows you that it was quite a while ago, as I don't even think you can buy CD players anymore! But you can buy a small portable radio for less than £20, and that, with some headphones, would be a great hospital gift.

Lean on me

A really useful thing to be is the friend who organises the other friends. When someone you love is ill, it is often all you can do to get dressed in the morning, let alone start drawing up a list of who's doing what, and it is such a relief if someone takes this on. You may wonder if you are the right person to do this, as everyone tends to think there's another 'better' friend, but trust me, organising other people into a rota for visiting, cooking meals or driving to hospital, or just rounding up a bunch of mates to give your pal a night out, will be very welcome. And it's a small thing, but finding out when a friend's birthday is and reminding everyone to send cards is much appreciated!

Competitive illness syndrome

It is very easy to get so wrapped up in your own problems that you become totally uninterested in everyone else's. This absorption is not healthy, and you must try to keep things in perspective and appreciate that everyone has their own struggles. My thoughts sometimes ran along the lines of, 'Well, I don't know what on earth she's worried about, she might have her ill parents to look after, but try having a husband in hospital for 11 months!'

But someone with an ill child could well be thinking the same about me, and truly, there isn't a hierarchy to illnesses, we all just need to try and share compassion. It can be helpful when friends let you talk and talk, but I would advise almost forcing yourself to keep it within a fixed time frame, before asking them about their own lives and making sure you listen to them properly. Not wallowing too much in your own worries will do you a lot of good. When I was really down, I found that hearing about other people's challenges actually made me feel much better than hearing about people who were having a great time, which made me envious and miserable!

Empathy is a great thing, but if you are the one listening to someone talking about an illness, proceed with caution before adding your own anecdotes. Everyone needs to feel that their own life is special, and adding in 'Oh that sounds like my grandma' can come across as devaluing a unique experience. I lost count of the times people said of encephalitis, 'that's like Alzheimer's', and it made me want to scream, 'I'm not remotely interested in whether it's like Alzheimer's or not; how is that relevant to me?'

Handle with care

Almost exactly three years since Alan went into hospital, early in the new year, a painter arrives to quote for decorating Sam's bedroom. 'Sorry I didn't get back to you sooner,' he says as soon as he comes in, 'but my dad's just gone into hospital.' His face has the bewildered look of someone to whom something utterly catastrophic has happened and he can't quite understand how everyday life is still carrying on. Every second sentence he mentions it. 'I can get the paint for you, but things are a bit up in the air... Not too busy at the moment, although with my dad... Should be OK to start in a couple of weeks although...' He trails off. I tell him it's fine – to send me a quote when he has a moment, I'm not in a hurry.

I feel such a rush of recollection for that time in January 2017 when I too was walking through the world unable to comprehend how everyone else could be behaving as if things were normal. You feel like you want to say to everyone you meet, 'Please be nice to me, something awful has just happened, and I'm struggling to cope.' But you don't have a sign on you saying 'fragile', and of course, the world carries on regardless. The week Alan went into hospital, the windscreen-washer fluid ran out in my car, and because Alan had always done it for me, I didn't even know how to open the bonnet, let alone top it up. I couldn't think what to do, so I drove into our brilliant local garage with Madeleine, burst into tears and begged Mick to help me. He must have thought I was completely mad, but he just calmly sorted it out in about 30 seconds. It makes me laugh now, but I remember so vividly how distraught I felt over the smallest thing going wrong.

It was the same when my father-in-law died: our drain needed unblocking, and when the guy came, I was feeling extremely emotional, and I remember talking to him as if he was some sort of counsellor. Again, he was totally unfazed and very nice. People are, on the whole. You may not be wearing a sign that tells people to handle you with care, but I strongly recommend opening up and sharing what's on your mind when the opportunity arises. Making a connection and giving people the opportunity to say something kind to you rather than thinking 'Blimey, what's her problem?' makes the world a far better place.

Chapter Ten

REASONS TO BE CHEERFUL

How to be Happy in Hard Times

The power of laughter

I HEAR THE BESTSELLING IRISH author Marian Keyes speaking on Radio 2's *Jeremy Vine* show, and what she says really strikes a chord with me. She is talking about when her father was seriously ill in hospital, and she and her mother were desperately trying to get him to take a tablet. Just when they think he has finally swallowed it, he spits it back into the glass of water. Suddenly, amidst the intense frustration:

> Out of nowhere, she and I were in absolute convulsions, helpless with laughter, we laughed and laughed until tears ran down our faces and every time it seemed like the bout had run its course, all we had to do was make eye contact and we were off again.

She goes on to say that:

> Afterwards, despite the fact that Dad still hadn't taken his medication, we felt better than we had for ages. Our mood was elevated, in fact we were positively giddy, and even our muscles felt relaxed.

I know so well what she means when she says that 'one of the things that makes us human is that we use laughter as a survival mechanism'. Weirdly, the darkest days can provide the funniest moments, and I'm sure she is right to think that it is our own body's way of coping. Humour is vital for getting you through the horrible times. Whether it's black humour, slapstick silliness or smiling bravely through your tears, laughter is one of the most powerful weapons in our armoury. Anyone who knows a medical student will have heard about the many jokes and pranks that help them get through the harrowing training, and one of the many reasons the brilliant *This is Going to Hurt* by Adam Kay has been so successful is that it is side-splittingly, eye-poppingly hilarious. Humour and illness may not seem like obvious partners, but they absolutely are.

Why are there no aspirins in the jungle?[1]

Our own moment for hysterical laughter comes a few days after Alan has come round from the coma. He is breathing on his own again, and he can talk, but his brain is so scrambled that he cannot think of the words for everyday things. The doctors

---

1   Because the parrots eat 'em all.

hold up a pen, a notebook, a cup, and ask him what they are, but he just shakes his head in bafflement. The feeding tube has been taken out, and he's learning to eat by himself. Since we're there at supper time, the nurse suggests that Sam and I help him to spoon up the meat, potatoes, gravy and veg. We're chatting away to him as we do this, and Sam says, 'Dad, what are those vegetables called that you're eating now? Those little round green things.' He looks at them carefully. 'P...' he says. We nod. 'P...P...P.' 'Yes, that's right,' we say, willing him on. 'P...?' Suddenly he smiles triumphantly. 'Parrots!' he exclaims.

Vlad the Impaler

Relearning the names of our large family is another cause of confusion for Alan's poor disconnected brain and a source of hilarity for us. Like many parents, he has often previously interchanged his children's names – to be fair, Lucy, Izzy and Maddy as well as Simon and Sam are easy to muddle up – but now it is on a whole new level. One day I ask him who is here with me, and he stares at Sam for many minutes before finally saying 'Vladimir?' We show him a photo of his niece Alison and nephew Andrew and ask if he knows who they are, to which he replies, 'Manuela and Konstanz.' Another day, I ask him if he can remember the really good news about Lucy and Craig. Their recent adoption of gorgeous baby George has brought us all such joy, and we've shown him lots of photos and videos. 'Remember?' I say. 'They've recently got someone new in their family. Someone small.' He stares at me, concentrating hard. 'A little...' he says. 'Yes,' I say encouragingly. 'A little...' His brow furrows. 'A little, a little...insect?' I decide not to tell Lucy that George's new grandpa thinks he's a caterpillar.

Old MacDonald had a farm

Once Alan learnt to speak properly again, we thought for a brief moment that his sanity had returned. But very quickly we realised that not knowing the names for things was actually the least of his problems. Despite having nothing wrong with his eyesight, his brain could not properly process what he saw, and converting that information into logical thought or sensible speech was impossible. At the time, it seemed as if he was hallucinating, which was disconcerting to say the least, but also funny.

One time, he looked at the man in the bed across the ward and said to us loudly, 'Why has that man got a big banana coming out of his nose?' The seriously ill gentleman in the bed opposite was, in fact, connected to an oxygen tube and probably didn't appreciate either Alan's comment or our quickly stifled laughter. Another time, he could see a patient's two bare feet peeping over the top of the rail at the end of a bed. He became convinced that they were two people, looking over the railing of a passing cruise ship! In fact, this belief that he was on a ship became more and more common, and he often remarked on how nice it was to be in the warm Caribbean. The blue curtains round the beds became the sea, and once he'd moved to a room where he could see out of a window, the view from ten floors up tricked his brain into thinking he was in an aeroplane. He would greet us as if we were on-board or in-flight visitors and rarely acknowledged that the preponderance of doctors, nurses and medical equipment would seem to indicate that he was, in fact, in hospital.

Then, for a long time, he thought he was on a farm and would frequently complain about how hard he had to work. Small movements just out of his line of vision convinced him that rabbits were hopping around him. One morning, he said to Simon that he had a sore throat, 'from shouting at all the animals'. When Simon queried the likelihood of this, he said patiently, as if Simon was not very bright, 'The animals in the field. They all escaped this morning. Four cows, two pigs, six horses. It took hours. You have no idea.'

Always look on the bright side

Children's books from a hundred years or so ago are full of protagonists who suffer from a life-changing or life-threatening illness. Saintly Beth with scarlet fever in *Little Women*, Katy with a broken back in *What Katy Did*, the bed-ridden Colin in *The Secret Garden*, blind sister Mary in the *Little House on the Prairie* series and Clara in her wheelchair in *Heidi*; many classic novels feature illness. Suffering from a serious childhood ailment was undoubtably a far more likely occurrence back then; however, 'sick lit', as the *Daily Mail* unhelpfully dubs it, is still a genre popular with young readers. Bestselling examples include the teen novels *The Fault in Our Stars* and *Before I Die*, both of which feature children suffering from cancer. Perhaps, the authors aim to help young people going through similar afflictions.

However, writers are undoubtably also using this literary meme as a way of encouraging readers to face adversity with courage and fortitude. The most famous exponent of this is probably *Pollyanna*, eponymous heroine of the 1913 novel by Eleanor H. Porter. An orphan (like so many stars of children's literature), she develops 'The Glad Game' as a way of coping with life's trials: 'The game was just to find something about everything to be glad about – no matter what 'twas.' She first discovers it as a way of dealing with the disappointment of not getting a doll for

Christmas when the missionary charity box gives her a pair of children's crutches. And she realises that she can be glad about that because she doesn't need the crutches. She spends most of the novel cheerfully helping all the neighbourhood pessimists to perk themselves up a bit. Things come to a climax when Polly-anna is hit by a car and nearly dies. After being glad that at least she isn't ill, because 'broken legs get well and lifelong-invalids don't', she is given the news that she is in fact paralysed from the waist down. Even Pollyanna finds this news devastating and sobs, 'Why, if I can't walk, how am I ever going to be glad for – anything?' Sadness descends on the entire community. 'To think that now – never again would that cheery little voice proclaim the gladness of some everyday experience. It seemed unbelievable, impossible, cruel. In kitchen and sitting rooms, and over backyard fences, women talked of it and wept openly. On street corners and in store lounging-places the men talked too and wept – though not quite so openly.' Finally, Pollyanna realises that she can, in spite of everything, still be glad. First, because of the positive effect she discovers she has had on all the other people in the town, and second, because she recognises that at least she can be grateful that she has had the use of her legs for the previous 11 years of her life. Of course, right at the end of the novel, a cure is miraculously found, and Pollyanna learns to walk again. 'Oh, I'm so glad! I'm glad for everything. Why, I'm glad now I lost my legs for a while, for you never, never know how perfectly lovely legs are till you haven't got them.'

Most readers these days will find the virtuous Pollyanna pretty insufferable. Tiny Tim with his leg braces and crutch chirruping 'God bless us, everyone' at the end of *A Christmas Carol* is equally irritating. But nonetheless, a fictional character who radiates optimism in the bleakest times is undeniably a powerful symbol.

The crucified victims in *Life of Brian* cheerfully exhorting us to 'Always look on the bright side of life', even though 'life's a piece of shit, when you look at it' were not very long ago regarded as highly blasphemous and controversial. Yet nowadays, that Monty Python song is frequently asked for on the radio by those going through tough times and is the number-one song requested on funeral playlists.

Turn that frown upside down

Without being too much like Pollyanna, I think adopting a 'find the positive in the negative' attitude can be a really helpful way to tackle illness. If you have undergone CBT (cognitive behavioural therapy), you will know that it is partly a matter of training your brain to think along different lines to the ones it has got used to using. The more you do this, the more it will become a habit. For me, the first way to make myself feel less sorry for myself was to think what would have happened if Alan had had his first seizure 48 hours earlier. Instead of being in a carpeted room with me there to break his sudden fall, he would have been at the wheel of his large car, driving five of us at 80mph down the fast lane of the motorway. The consequences of that first collapse would have been almost unimaginably worse, and I didn't have to be Pollyanna to feel that it was something to be glad about and grateful for.

And according to a 30-year study, being optimistic can actually help you live longer. Researchers in an American study (2019), based on over 70,000 people, found that the most optimistic men and women had, on average, an 11–15% longer lifespan and 50–70% greater odds of reaching 85 years old than the least optimistic groups. Optimism was defined as a 'general expectation that good things will happen or believing that the future will be favourable'.

However, I think it is important to differentiate between trying to be positive and believing that positive thinking will beat the illness. Susan Sontag, in her ground-breaking book *Illness as Metaphor*, challenged the idea that it was important for the patient to 'fight' cancer or try to 'will' themselves better. Sontag was herself suffering from cancer when she wrote her book, as was Barbara Ehrenreich, author of *Bright-Sided: How the Relentless Promotion of Positive Thinking Has Undermined America*. She too disputed the belief that by being upbeat you could improve your own health and wellbeing, dismissing it as 'pseudoscientific flapdoodle'.

Personally, I feel that although being optimistic may not affect the outcome of an illness, it will have a major effect on how you and your family cope with it, which is almost as important.

Oh no he isn't!

Alan's time in intensive care was a surreal slipstream between life and death when the hospital was both a place of succour and a place of dread. But one morning, as Madeleine and I walk down the corridor, we notice lots of jolly new posters, urging all staff to COME ALONG TO THE HOSPITAL PANTO MEETING! It is clear that there is going to be a pantomime in February, staged by, and presumably for the entertainment of, the many staff working in the large hospital.

It gives Mads and me exactly the same thrill as you get when, as a child, you discover that your teachers actually have a life outside school. We clutch each other, spluttering with laughter as we imagine all the NHS workers – from the grumpy receptionist to the angelic ICU nurses, to the serious and unsmiling neurologists – all breaking into song, waving 'jazz hands', high-kicking in a chorus line. Then, we overhear Dr Morven asking another doctor, 'Are you coming along to the panto meeting tonight?', which sets us off into even more hysterics. Dr Morven is a bit of a dish and we cannot decide whether he will be playing the romantic lead or if he has a secret life as a pantomime dame. Sadly, Alan leaves that hospital before we get any answers. But our fevered imaginings and silly speculations help to get us through a terrible week.

Funny things and fun things

Aside from trying to find funny things to cheer us up while we're in the hospital, we get better at making sure we find fun things to do outside the hospital as well. It's easy when you are stressed just to exist in a bubble of worry, but you must make yourself do other things.

We discover new places to eat near the hospital and have impromptu meals out in cosy restaurants and wintery drinks in sunny pub gardens. Eating tasty, nurturing food is proven to have a major effect on your mood, and I find that taking an hour every evening to cook a proper meal helps me to relax and makes us all feel better.

My book-club girls – Annie, Jane S, Jane O, Louise, Maria and Susanna – as well as giving me much emotional support, provide very welcome wicked humour. Other friends take me out and make me laugh. Sam and I go to the cinema and revel in the escapism of the Marvel universe and *Star Wars*. I start to pop into some of the clothes shops on the way home from the hospital; sometimes I go out for lunch rather than eating a sandwich in Alan's room. In short, we discover that life goes on and that it is possible to balance uncertainty and sadness with genuine fun.

The cheer that a compliment can bring

One sunny Monday in spring, I arrive in a T-shirt dress that I bought from Primark on my way home the Friday before. I bought it to cheer myself up, thinking that its jolly red and blue stripes would be life enhancing, but now it feels too tight, too short and just wrong. I'm definitely wearing the wrong knickers; the fabric makes my tummy look wobbly. Alan is not in a good mood, there is nothing to learn from the doctors today and I make it a short visit. I stand waiting for the lift, tugging a bit at my dress, feeling self-conscious.

A tall, stylish woman, younger than me, gets out of the lift and immediately says, 'Oh, I *love* your dress. That looks really great on you.' I am amazed. 'I see you here a lot,' she continues, 'and you always look good. Always making an effort. That's good.' I am ridiculously flattered and crazily pleased. 'Thanks,' I say. 'Thanks a lot.' 'I mean it,' she says. 'You look good.' That one remark improves my whole day by about 400%. In fact, it improves my whole week. It makes me realise how much a compliment can lift you up, and I resolve to give some out myself. It also makes me appreciate the value of connecting with strangers – I have never even noticed her before – and I make up my mind to look around me, be more aware of other people in the hospital and smile at them.

And he drove the fastest milk cart in the west

One morning, when Alan is in the neurology ward, I arrive at his bedside to find a little knot of keenie-beanie medical students clustered around him. Throughout the five months Alan was in this hospital, we all found it very heartening to hope that his experience would add to the general medical knowledge available. 'Can we ask your husband some questions?'

Even now, several years later, quite experienced medical professionals – from GPs to therapists – find it hard to comprehend that the answers they are going to get from someone with a brain injury are more than likely to be nonsense.

One fresh-faced medic asks Alan what his job is, and without missing a beat, Al says, 'A milkman. I'm a milkman.' He then proceeds to explain in some detail what this entails, where his daily round is, how many pints he delivers, the fact that it's an enjoyable job because it's outdoors and he meets lots of different people and so on. After about five minutes of this highly convincing baloney, the student turns to me, an earnest expression on his face. 'That's right, is it Mrs Jessop?' And through my giggles, I explain that no, no it isn't, that my husband is not – and never has been – a milkman! To me, the thought of him pootling around like Benny Hill's Ernie seems totally ridiculous. To the medic, this unshaven, chatty old man in a hospital gown could be anyone.

I think: where on *earth* did that confabulation come from? Did a nurse mention milk maybe? Did one of the machines sound like a milk float? Or in fact, does he secretly want to be a milkman? Sharing moments like this with the family over supper lightened up some very dark days, and the fact that brain illnesses can be comedic is a huge contradiction in terms. Seeing someone you love talking nonsense is, at best, disconcerting, at worst, terrifying. But I think to deny that it is also incredibly funny is to deny what makes us human.

Many people who've had an elderly relation with a urine infection have had similar experiences. The bacteria in the urinary tract makes sufferers delirious, and I remember my 94-year-old father-in-law once ringing me up at 4am to tell me that he was trapped at Victoria train station with a large brass band marching round him, and could I please tell him how he should get back home to Croydon! Eventually, I managed to convince him that he was at home in his bed, but it was a close-run thing.

Keep on truckin'

Once Alan is well enough to watch TV in the day room, the temporary effects of this on his brain provide even more entertainment. The draw for the next round of the FA Cup is enough to convince him that the entire Chelsea team will be arriving imminently in his bedroom, and he needs to get ready to greet them. A while later, he watches the Chelsea vs Spurs match at Wembley on TV with Sam, but despite the fact that he is sitting in his pyjamas and slippers on a hospital chair, he becomes increasingly certain that he is, in fact, at Wembley, cheering on the Blues. As the match draws to a close, he starts fretting about the traffic and keeps getting up and looking for his car keys, telling Sam that they need to get going or 'It will be a nightmare on the North Circular.' The funniest thing is that, by now, his speech is pretty normal, and he always delivers these gems with no indication that he's talking nonsense.

One afternoon, while drinking a cup of tea and watching a programme about trucks, I tell Alan that Simon (who has an office-based job in the centre of town) will be in to visit later that evening. Without missing a beat, he says that I must 'Tell him that he needs to be very careful driving his lorry over the Severn Bridge, there are very strong winds today.'

Be more sisu

'Sisu' is a Finnish word that doesn't really have a direct translation but encompasses extreme perseverance and dignity in the face of adversity. A mixture of grit, determination and courage, it briefly took over as the Scandi 'it trend' following 'hygge'. Hygge, which means a sort of snuggly cosiness, is virtually impossible to achieve in hospital, but sisu is much more like it. The word originates from the Finnish word 'sisus', which literally means 'guts', and was embraced by a country looking for positive images of itself when Finland became independent from Russia in 1917; strengthening the idea to the Finns that there was something special about them. *The New York Times* ran an article in 1940 with the headline 'Sisu: A Word that Explains Finland', referring to the bombing of the 'Winter War' of 1939–40 when Finland was attacked by the much superior Soviet army but managed to mount a resistance to remain independent.

Believing that you are special and that you are a survivor is undoubtably a good frame of mind to adopt, whether you are the patient or the carer. I think sisu is particularly useful, as it does not mean pretending that life is rosy; instead, it is more about accepting things are difficult, but getting on with them anyway. The Japanese have a similar word, 'ganbaru' (or 頑張る), which roughly means slogging tenaciously through the tough times.

Reasons to be cheerful

A year or so after Alan has come home, Paul, an old work friend of Alan's, emails me out of the blue to ask after his health. He says he doesn't know why, but a favourite song has just popped into his head when he thinks about him. The song is Ian Dury's *Reasons to be Cheerful*.

I email Paul straight back to say that this has always been a favourite song of Al's as well, and that he is chuffed by both the email and the connection. The moment lifts all three of us.

Ian Dury had plenty of reasons *not* to be cheerful, since he was disabled from childhood polio, which left him with a paralysed left arm and leg. But he had a thoroughly robust attitude to both his own disability and illness. When dying of cancer, he was asked by a journalist whether he ever felt sorry for himself and replied, 'No. Sorry for yourself is for wankers, innit?' and 'Look up sympathy in the dictionary, and you'll find it comes between shit and syphilis, ha, ha!' In 1981, Dury's song *Spasticus Autisticus* (which he wrote to show his disdain for the International Year of Disabled Persons, believing it to be deeply patronising) was banned by the BBC, but in 2012, thanks to hugely changed attitudes to disability, it was used in the opening ceremony for the London Paralympic Games.

Accentuate the positive

Lucy O'Donnell decided to turn the devasting news that she had incurable breast cancer into something constructive and optimistic. Reviewers have praised her inspiring book *Cancer is My Teacher*, for the way she has managed to turn a terrible disease into a positive experience. She has discovered not just how to survive, but also how to retain an astonishing appetite for life despite her awful circumstances. Lucy's message of not just surviving but thriving is one that I can relate to. I hear another cancer survivor called Toni Crews talking on the radio. Tumours in her tear glands meant she had to have her left eye removed, but she has decided to combat the horrendousness of this with making and wearing fantastically colourful eye patches. She now sells them on her website Bling-K of An Eye to help other people who have to wear an eyepatch feel more confident. She says that the biggest lesson she has learnt is that 'time is short and life is precious, you should do what makes you happy' and that 'positivity is a huge help'. Her favourite mantra is a quote from Eleanor Roosevelt who said 'We gain strength, and courage, and confidence by each experience in which we really stop to look fear in the face...we must do that which we think we cannot.'

Finding the funny

Once Alan is in a Brain Rehab Centre on the other side of town, we realise that he will have to learn to use his mobile again in order to contact us. Slightly to our surprise, most of the time this works OK. I have taken all the contacts off his phone apart from close family, and muscle memory seems to kick in when it comes to pressing the right combination of buttons to make a call. But many of our conversations have an utterly surreal tone as he still has no idea where he is and definitely no idea where we are!

In fact, this marks a growing realisation that however awful Alan's brain damage is, it is OK to laugh at it sometimes – and it is also OK to use it to our advantage. Sometimes, when he rings, he is very scared and worried, and that is really hard to hear. Other times though, he talks cheerfully about how well the Sales Conference is going in Australia, and how he has just seen a kangaroo jumping past his window. And I realise that it's OK to prefer the conversations with the happy, loopier Alan than the saner, sadder Alan. I also realise that I can say I'll be in to see him 'soon' or even 'this afternoon' even if that's not true. He won't remember, and it will cheer him up to hear it.

This comes in especially handy when Izzy, Madeleine, Sam and I go away for a much-needed break. Talking to me always cheers him up and it doesn't matter that I'm hundreds of miles away. Even nowadays, his brain doesn't always process the information around him properly, which can be entertaining. A couple of summers ago, we were staying in a villa in France, and when I told him it was time to get in the car, he walked directly towards it. The only problem was that this took him straight into the swimming pool. Luckily, he was standing near the shallow end.

Only connect

Alan and I are sitting on uncomfortable chairs, in a circle, at a meeting run by Headway, a brilliant charity that supports people with brain injuries. Most people there are with a partner, but one young man has come by himself. He starts talking in broken English about how glad he is to have found this group and how much it means to him. He lives alone, and my eyes fill with tears as he describes how difficult he is finding life and how hard it is to keep going. He tells us that, honestly, if it wasn't for coming to these sessions, he doesn't know how he would cope. It hits me like a sledgehammer that illness is a thousand times sadder if you are going through it alone. It makes me realise that although Alan may soon be getting to the point where he doesn't need (or want) the support of this group, maybe we need to keep attending in order to bolster others.

There has been quite a bit of research into the effects of loneliness. Studies (Holt-Lunstad *et al.*, 2015) show that lacking social connections can be as damaging to your health as smoking 15 cigarettes a day and increases your risk of dying by 26%. Loneliness is associated with an increased risk of developing heart disease and stroke, puts you at greater risk of cognitive decline and depression and is predictive of suicide. If you become ill, therefore, the very worst thing you can do is go through it alone. And it must surely be the case that having people around you can help your recovery. When you are ill or recovering, you may not feel remotely like joining a choir, a worship group, a club or any other social gathering but it is likely to be one of the best things you could do.

A friendly face

Finding company once you're recovering at home is one thing, but perhaps even more important is getting some company while you're actually in hospital. According to research carried out by the Royal Voluntary Service (RVS) (2019), 40% of patients on UK hospital wards get no visitors at all. The RVS have a wide range of hospital volunteer opportunities and there is lots of information on their website.[2] Christine Thorne, who volunteers at the Aberdeen Royal Infirmary, said, 'It makes me sad to think there are people with no one at all to come and see them. Hospitals can

2   https://volunteering.royalvoluntaryservice.org.uk/volunteering-in-hospitals

be a scary place at the best of times, more so if you don't have a friendly face to help you through it.'

Perhaps, when we are visiting a friend or relation, we should all get better at pausing on the way out to have a chat with another patient. And this might be even better if you have a child with you. I remember, when visiting my great aunt in a nursing home, how the other residents' eyes would light up with joy if I had small children with me, and how just bringing a toddler or baby onto the premises seemed to spread a little happiness.

Top ten tips for being happy in hardship

- Connect with people. Chat to the other patients on a ward.
- Look for laughter. It could be a funny book, a joke on your phone or finding the black humour in your situation. Laughing is good for you.
- Be interested in the lives of the people looking after you. This will make the whole process more human and less clinical.
- Try and find something to be glad about.
- Cultivate resilience, grit and courage.
- Remind yourself that optimists live longer.
- Spread some compliments around. They cost nothing and make everyone feel better.
- Accentuate the positive and read about other people who have. Do not read sad books.
- Force yourself to put a brave face on things and eventually it will become second nature.
- Treat yourself.

Chapter Eleven

CRAZY FOR YOU

The Mental Health of the Patient and the Carer

O, let me not be mad

KING LEAR'S LINES 'O, let me not be mad, not mad, sweet heaven! I would not be mad. Keep me in temper. I would not be mad' resonate with most of us, and suffering some sort of brain-related ailment is an almost universal fear. And whether you are the patient or the family, any illness brings with it enormous potential for depression and despair.

A review of 'The Prevalence of Depression in General Hospital Inpatients' (2018) revealed that 'depression frequently accompanies physical illness', which was 'important because it is associated with worse physical symptoms and a poorer quality of life'. Another study (2000) showed that patients suffering from poor mental health 'spend more time in hospital and are less likely to adhere to medical treatments'. And if your illness is related to a brain injury in the first place, the statistics are even worse. One study (1981) showed that survivors of a brain injury are 57% more likely than people who haven't had a brain injury to suffer from depression, and their partners, 79% more likely.

The Mental Health Foundation say that 'people who live with a long-term condition are also likely to experience mental ill-health, such as depression and anxiety'. Their research (2011) reveals that 'more than 15 million people in the UK live with one or more long-term conditions and more than 4 million also have a mental health problem'. This is a hugely important issue, and possibly one that hospitals and doctors don't deal with as well as they might – usually because the resources just aren't available.

The lunatics have taken over the asylum

I had never heard of encephalitis before Alan got it and often recall the doctor telling me that not so very long ago, his condition would have been diagnosed as 'unexplained madness'. And its treatment would have been, at best, experimental, and at worst, brutal. With no small degree of irony, one of Alan's favourite books and films was *One Flew Over the Cuckoo's Nest*, Ken Kesey's 1962 novel set in a US psychiatric hospital, which is both a passionate roar in defence of individuality and a damning indictment of mental wards as instruments of oppression.

One of the first countries to build asylums, the UK was also one of the first countries to turn away from them as the main way of looking after the mentally ill, marking a shift towards care in the community. But the crime writer P. D. James, who worked in the NHS and whose husband was a long-term patient in a mental hospital, observed in 1999 that community care 'could be described more accurately as the absence of care in a community still largely resentful or frightened of mental illness'.

A short timeline of mental health care in Britain

- The most famous of all mental hospitals is Bedlam (the nickname for the Bethlem Royal Hospital), which was founded in London in 1247. It wasn't founded as a mental hospital, but by the mid-1400s had become a specialist institution for the 'confinement of the insane'. By the 1500s, the term 'bedlam' had entered everyday speech to signify a state of madness and chaos. Despite its large reputation, it remained small for centuries; in 1620 it had just 24 patients.
- In 1676, Bedlam moved to a much bigger building. The hospital allowed visitors with no connection to the inmates as a way of raising income, and this display of madness as public entertainment and instruction has often been considered one of its most shocking features. It was the only public mental institution in England until well into the 1800s. Today, it is a research and treatment centre.
- The Madhouses Act of 1774 was the first UK legislation to address mental health. Privately funded lunatic asylums were widely established during the 19th century, and the 1845 Lunacy Act was an important landmark in the treatment of the mentally ill, as it changed their status to patients who required treatment.
- The 1890 Lunacy Act placed an obligation on local

authorities to maintain institutions for the mentally ill, and by 1938, 131,000 patients were in mental hospitals in England and Wales, with 13,000 in Scotland.

- Mental health services were not integrated with physical health services when the NHS was established in 1948, and shortages of money, staff and buildings were widespread. The 1950s and 60s also saw an explosion in the treatment of mental illness with mood-altering drugs, such as the widely prescribed anti-anxiety drug Valium.

- In 1961 the Conservative Minister for Health was so appalled by what he witnessed on his visits to the asylums that he called for their closure and their replacement by wards in general hospitals. The majority of mental health care is now provided by the NHS, assisted by the private and the voluntary sectors.

- Most of the institutions created by the Victorians are gone and, as a result, there has been a spectacular decline in the number of beds available for psychiatric patients. In the 1950s, there were approximately 150,000 beds available for mental health patients in England; in 2017, there were around 18,500.

Today, at any one time, some seven million people in England and Wales over the age of 16 (one in six of the adult population) are suffering from a significant psychiatric problem. At least a third of all families have a member who will at some stage be mentally ill. And as a society, we are struggling to cope. Data compiled for the BBC by NHS Digital showed that between 2011–12 and 2015–16 the number of patients attending A&E units with psychiatric problems rose by nearly 50%. As Christie Watson writes in her book *The Language of Kindness*, 'Patients who are suffering from severe mental health disorder have an unacceptable wait in A&E and the environment is completely inappropriate for those who are already vulnerable and disorientated.'

All in the mind?

When Alan first became ill, I felt it was somehow very important that everyone should know that the damage to his brain was caused by a 'proper' illness, by something detectable and measurable on a brain scan. I hated the thought that people might think it was due to what used to be called 'a nervous breakdown'. This was partly because I hoped that if there was a physical cause then it would be simpler to treat, but I confess, it was also due to the stigma around mental health. To some extent, my 'if you can see it, you can cure it' theory is true. We have all heard of cases where a brain tumour is eliminated, and a person miraculously returns to full health.

But there is still a colossal amount that the scientists don't yet know about how the brain recovers after trauma, whether it's physical or mental, and the differences between psychological and physiological brain damage are not always distinct. The doctors talk about brain 'plasticity', which means how well a brain can change and adapt. Scientists know that your brain can't grow new cells to replace those that are damaged. But there is still much debate around the question of how well a brain can make new connections between the cells that it still has – how well it can 'rewire' itself.

We often used the analogy of a road. The synapses that connect different parts of the brain should be smooth and unbroken so that the thoughts can whizz along them speedily. But if they are damaged, it's like trying to drive along a bumpy track full of potholes, and a better option would be to use an alternative route.

A human brain certainly can increase its capacity. A baby's brain grows to reach half its adult size within three months and 80% of its adult size in two years. And its development is directly influenced by what it learns – nurture rather than nature. But how much an adult brain can physically change and what might cause a change is much debated. The damage to Alan's brain could be viewed on an MRI, but the things that the doctors can't see are also relevant. Even when there is no measurable evidence of brain change after illnesses such as depression, it may be because we don't yet have the science to find it.

And the line between mental illness and mental health is a fuzzy one. Encephalitis, a stroke, a tumour, Alzheimer's and dementia are all things that can cause brain damage. Those who have suffered from stress, an eating disorder, depression, anxiety or OCD might not describe their brains as 'damaged', but whatever the reason why a brain is malfunctioning, there is good scientific evidence that the same things will help or hinder its recovery. Rest, routine, company, tranquillity, positivity and fresh air are good. And loneliness, incarceration, noise, anger, unkindness and hopelessness are not.

'She's not usually like this'

Early on, I arrive in the high-dependency unit to hear raucous shouting. An elderly woman is trying to get out of bed and is being restrained by the nurses. She is yelling furiously, using all manner of swear words without any care as to who hears her. I am uncomfortable on her behalf, sorry for the staff, concerned for the other patients. It is horrible. Then a woman about my age comes in with a cup of tea; it's her daughter. She looks deeply embarrassed. 'Oh god,' she says. 'It's awful isn't it? She's not usually like this, I didn't even know Mum knew those words. She would hate it if she knew that people were seeing her like this. She's such a gentle person.' I am ashamed to say that, at the time, I didn't believe her. I just couldn't imagine that someone's personality could change so completely, and although I smiled sympathetically at the woman, inside I was making my own judgements.

A month later, I am in a different hospital, watching my own kind, mild-mannered husband swearing vehemently at the lovely occupational therapist (OT) who is not allowing him to leave the ward. 'F**k off!' he screams. 'Just f**k off, all of you, f**k right off.' Earlier in the week, we were horrified to see him roaring at another nurse who was sitting at a laptop, which he believed to be a TV. 'Why don't you just get off your fat arse and let me watch that telly?' he bellowed. We were mortified; all we could do was apologise, tell ourselves the staff must be used to it and try and find some humour in the situation. By now, Alan has been moved to his own room, with round-the-clock one-to-one care from registered mental health nurses (RMNs), but the next week, the self-locking mechanism to the ward door is broken, and all visitors must come in another way. To my horror, and acute shame, I find out it is Alan who has smashed it. Then, worst of all, one morning the enormous plate-glass window in his room is splintered right across, the long cracks temporarily mended with black gaffer tape, giving the room the appearance of a prison cell. Alan has pushed a drip stand into it.

The violence of illness is extremely frightening. I discover that ferocious mood swings are common after a brain injury, and it helps a lot just to know this. I was very moved by Alison Murdoch's *Bed 12*, an emotional and powerful book about a woman whose husband also had encephalitis. But one sentence I have an issue with is when she says 'I'm proud of the fact that there is no anger or aggression in him, just puzzlement and deep confusion'. I now know that someone who is ill cannot control their own mind, and rage in the mentally ill is not something to be ashamed of.

Losing your mind

Even worse than the furious hostility is the disturbing sensation that Alan is turning into someone else. Perhaps the most terrifying of all mental illnesses is schizophrenia, and for a couple of months, his ability to switch between two personalities is genuinely frightening. For a while, he refuses to believe that I am Catherine, and keeps asking for, 'not this wife, the other one'. Even more upsetting for me is the fact that although we have been married for 23 years, he sometimes thinks that maybe I am his first wife, the mother of my two stepchildren, Lucy and Simon. Sometimes he is unable to decide which I am and says that I am speaking with one voice but looking like another, and please can I stop it. Sometimes he doesn't know who I am at all and shouts at me to leave and bring back the real Catherine. I find this incredibly upsetting and often leave the ward in tears. The worst thing is that when it happens, I never know when the 'glitch' will end. For my own sanity, I need to feel he is 'back to normal' before I leave, but of course, his brain doesn't work to my schedule. Much later, I read that this delusion is called 'Cap-gras syndrome' after the psychiatrist who identified it. It occurs where the brain tries to make sense of the fact that someone looks familiar but doesn't feel familiar, so it concludes that they must be an imposter.

The Brain Injury Rehabilitation Centre

Once Alan has had the plasma exchange and the Rituximab, the conversation begins to turn to what will happen next. I am coming to terms with the fact that he is not remotely 'recovered' and panicking about how he could possibly live at home. He is trying to escape on a regular basis, never knows where he is and sometimes doesn't know who we are. He is also in poor physical shape, not able to walk far (hardly surprising since he has been lying in bed for most of the last five months), very wobbly and often dribbling. I am finding it hard to cope with the idea that medical science has now done everything it can, and although he is working daily with an OT, I am not sure I believe that it is making any difference.

The senior OT tells me that they are planning to move Alan to a rehabilitation centre, which is good news. But I am taken aback when they give me the news that the best one is right over on the other side of the city. It will mean that he will no longer be 20 minutes away, but instead, the trip to see him will take closer to two hours. Which will make visiting much harder. But when they talk about the alternatives, I can see from their expressions that there are 'good' rehab units and ones that are not so good. Not for the first time, I appreciate what skilled hands Alan is in and understand that the level of care he is getting is not available for everyone who needs it.

Into the unknown

Our transfer from the hospital to the rehab centre is not auspicious. We are supposed to leave in the morning, but as is always the case, being discharged and waiting for all the medication to be prepared takes hours. Then there is another lengthy wait for a hospital taxi. Alan is agitated and tense. He doesn't understand what is happening or where he is going, and unfortunately, it turns out that the nurse who accompanies us and the taxi driver are almost as confused as he is. The traffic from west to east is terrible, and when we arrive it is early evening.

The driver peers anxiously at both his satnav and the road signs and eventually pulls up in front of a large hospital. 'Finally!' The nurse smiles and starts getting out. 'Wait a minute,' I say. 'This doesn't look right.' I Google the address on my phone, and sure enough, we are at the wrong hospital, although it has a similar name. The Brain Injury Rehabilitation Centre is one-and-a-half miles away. I am determined not to let Alan pick up on my anxiety, but I do wonder what would have happened if I hadn't been there. Would the nurse and Alan have wandered forever around the streets looking for help? When we finally do arrive at the correct address, it looks closed. The nurse and I stand at the front door pressing buzzers for ages. I will discover, during the six months that Alan stays here, that this is entirely the norm, and the Brain Rehab Centre is as impossible for visitors to get into as it is for patients to get out of. Frequently, we and other families will be standing at these doors for ten minutes or more, with the inmates waving to us from windows or chatting through the wire fence as we wait for a member of staff to appear. On that first evening, a small bespectacled man finally appears and leads us into a tiny waiting room. By now, Alan is off the scale with exhaustion, but the doctor in charge has a long questionnaire to fill in. The nurse who has come with us has never met Alan before, and after a frustrating ten minutes of her not knowing any of the answers to the questions, we agree that she may as well return to the hospital and I can speak for Alan. I am concerned that he has missed supper, so I insist that a sandwich and a cup of tea are found as the doctor starts filling in forms. Eventually, he leads us to Alan's room. It is small and dark, with a strong smell of disinfectant. Alan turns to me looking terrified. 'This isn't my room,' he says. 'I'm not staying here.' After five months of cheery familiar staff and brightly lit wards, this may be one of the best brain rehab units in the country, but it doesn't feel like it. The only good thing is that, by now, Alan is so tired that I know he will go straight to sleep.

I help him get into the little bed, with its dark green sheets and rustling plastic mattress cover. There is no bedside light, so I have to turn off the overhead light as I leave, and the heavy door has an automatic closer, so he is now in pitch-black darkness. I manage to find another member of staff and plead with her to look after him, explaining that he will have no idea where he is, how to find the door, the toilet, anything. She is nice, much nicer than the doctor, and explains that she can prop the door open and will check on him regularly. I leave, with the horrid sensation of having done as much as I can, and yet feeling that I haven't done nearly enough. I walk down the hill towards the bus stop with a heavy heart and begin the long bus and train journey home.

The Brain Rehab Centre is a good place, with kind and clever staff. Over the five months he is there, Alan makes progress. But like many care homes, it is hampered by an endless turnover of personnel. Three times, Alan gets to know his therapist well only for them to vanish overnight, replaced by another unfamiliar face. The long periods of time when no one is with him worry us. Staff in institutions sometimes refer to 'sundowning' – the phenomenon that means inmates appear to behave much more erratically in the evening – and we notice this too. During the day, there are visitors, classes, plenty of staff, meals, the opportunity to sit in the garden. After supper, which is served early, a gloomy evening stretches ahead, and Alan becomes visibly more agitated. And the undeniable and somewhat paradoxical truth about all places offering psychiatric care strikes us whenever we visit. Everyone else there is also mentally ill. This sometimes makes for a noisy, disturbing, frightening environment, not conducive to recovery.

Dark thoughts acknowledged

The talk from the Encephalitis Society[1] that I attend with Madeleine, about how families can build resilience following a brain injury, opens the floodgates to my pent-up feelings. It is hugely helpful for me to realise that others have these emotional thoughts too and to see them written down on a screen.

Difficult feelings

- Having to hold competing perspectives about the situation, e.g., 'He is gone' vs 'He's still here.' 'I'm glad she survived' vs 'I resent the burden.'
- Wanting to mourn but there is no death, grieving while the 'lost' person is still present.
- Doubting the fluctuating capabilities of the patient,

---

1   www.encephalitis.info

e.g., 'Are these behaviours really from the illness?' 'He can keep his temper when he wants to!'
- Finding it hard to adjust to the 'new' changed person when you are disrupted by momentary glimpses of the 'old' familiar person.
- Wanting your old life back and feeling anger that rehab can't provide that.
- Struggling with very dark emotions, e.g., 'I wish he'd died' – especially in the long term.
- Hating the unpredictability of patient outcomes and the resulting uncertainty in your own life.

Getting up and getting out

When someone is ill, and the future seems uncertain, the hardest part of any day can be getting out of bed. In the early days, there was a split second when I woke up before I remembered what had happened. But once reality came crashing into my thoughts, the temptation just to pull the covers over my head and stay under the duvet in the dark was massive. Staying in bed was a way of pretending that things weren't happening, of suspending time. And after 25 years of waking up next to someone you love, it is horrible waking up alone. But, as Barack Obama once said, 'The best way to not feel hopeless is to get up and do something.' I know that if you are suffering from depression, the worst thing can be staying in bed, and to try and stop myself sliding in that dangerous direction, I found tactics that worked for me.

How to get up

- Create a routine. I decided very quickly that I would go into hospital every morning. I didn't need to, and lots of people said, 'Oh be kind to yourself, have a lie-in and go in later.' But I found I was much happier if I made myself get up and out at the same time every day, as if it were a job. It stopped me feeling as if I were drifting and gave me purpose.
- Get some light into the room. This is hard to do in the winter, but just getting up and opening the curtains, even if it's grey, can make a big difference to your mood.
- Make sure you have something tasty in the house for breakfast. Even if you don't think of yourself as a breakfast person, it's much easier to get up when you know there is something nice to eat.
- Have a reason to get up. I had to make sure Sam was dressed and ready for school, but you could arrange to meet a friend for a walk or a coffee.
- Talk to yourself in the third person. This sounds weird, but psychologists say it can help to motivate you. So, rather than thinking 'I need to get up', I would say, 'Come on Catherine, time to get up. Let's go downstairs and put the kettle on. I know it's cold, but it will be warmer downstairs. Let's put the radio on and see what's going on in the world...' and so on.

Sinking

About a year after Alan has come home, I begin to feel myself sinking. The feeling almost seems to come out of the blue – nothing has got worse, but on the other hand, nothing has got better. Nothing dramatic has happened at all in fact, but the world suddenly feels unaccountably dreary. I am wading through mud, and I find myself weeping in inappropriate places and for no reason. I know that I need someone to help me, and my children have suggested as much, but oddly, although I have file after file of useful information for Alan, I can't think who to ask. I ring the Encephalitis Society, and they are lovely, but I don't feel as if I can keep ringing them up and crying. Then I find a fantastic organisation targeted at carers, but after an emotional conversation with a marvellous woman, she tells me gently that she won't be able to help me after this phone call, because I live in the wrong borough for her services. My own borough has a website but no phone number, or at least not one that anyone seems to be at the end of. I'm feeling more and more despairing.

But then, I notice on a leaflet for Integrated Neurological Services (a wonderful charity who have provided all sorts of therapeutic help for Al) that they also do counselling for carers. I cannot believe that I haven't seen this before. To my joy and gratitude, they can book me in for a block of ten 50-minute sessions with a trainee counsellor once a week. I find it incredibly helpful – just the excuse to talk about myself without feeling I am boring anyone is invaluable – and the advice gives me the momentum I need to keep going. The support of the counsellor gives me permission to see myself as a hero rather than a victim and also reminds me that when you are looking after someone with a serious illness or disability, it may well get harder, not easier.

Looking back on this time, I can appreciate that both friends and family – especially my children – were aware that I was struggling and trying desperately to help. Unfortunately, when your mind is fraught, you are not always in a place where you can accept support, and sadly, those closest to you may find it hardest to reach you.

Seeking to learn from my own experience, I think that if you are trying to help someone, it would be useful to write down what you want to say – including helpful contacts, references or phone numbers if you have them. A brain in turmoil can find it easier to process something in writing, and good, kind advice can easily be forgotten in the anxiety of the moment.

Caring for the carers

Looking after someone who is seriously ill puts a huge strain on your own wellbeing. Talking to friends and relations who are in a similar position confirms what I have already discovered, which is that although you will be in and out of your doctor's surgery all the time, this will do nothing for your own health! Of course, this is entirely understandable, as GPs are busy and need to focus on the problems in front of them, not all the subsidiary issues, but this can make you feel very unseen and resentful.

Recently, I took Alan to get a flu jab. On this occasion, we see a nurse rather than our GP, and although the appointment is for Alan, she puts two and two together when I explain the situation and asks about me. I am almost pathetically grateful and find myself welling up. 'What a terrible time you've had,' she says. 'How are you doing? It must be very difficult.' This is one of the very few times that a medical professional has touched on the emotional aspects of Alan's illness and how much it affects the carer as well as the patient. It makes an enormous difference, and I suddenly feel much less invisible.

It is important to remember that you can make your own appointment with your GP to discuss your mental health when you become a carer, and I would recommend that you do. There is also a lot of good practical advice about mental health on the Carers UK website.[2]

Recording to remember

When Alan was in the Brain Rehab Centre, the OTs suggested that he wrote a diary, and they tried it for a while, but Alan's writing was too unintelligible for it to be much use as neither he nor anyone else could read back what he had written! However, when he came home, Izzy discovered an app called Momento, which has been brilliant. This is a free app, which Alan uses on a tablet, but you can also use it on a phone. It makes it easy for you to write a diary entry each day and, best of all, you can add one photo to every entry. Alan cannot fill it in unaided, partly because despite having done it with me every day for three years, he still never remembers its existence! But he finds looking back at all the previous entries and the accompanying photos to be a positive experience.

I think many people really like the idea of keeping a diary but find the logistics of it too laborious. I would very much recommend a diary app, and if you are going through tough times with mental or physical health then it can be therapeutic to write

2   www.carersuk.org

things down. 'Journaling', as it's sometimes called, is enjoying a surge of popularity, tapping into the trends for mindfulness, gratitude and reflection, and as a result, there are lots of diary apps to choose from. Day One, Diarium, Journey, Penzu, Five Minute Journal and Daylio are some of the most popular.

Me time

Going into hospital every day or caring for someone at home is draining. People will often say to you that you must make more time for yourself. The problem is that if you are right in the middle of an exhausting experience, it is difficult to summon the energy to give yourself a proper break. Personally, I found the much-suggested hot bath surrounded by candles to be completely useless. Spending even more time in my own company, especially in a darkened room, just gave me more opportunity to dwell on dismal thoughts and worry about the future.

One day, my friend Alison rings from Chester. 'Antony and I are coming down,' she says. 'We've got tickets to the Hockney exhibition and you and Sam are coming with us.' The afternoon we spend at the gallery is life enhancing and life changing. As soon as we walk in, I can feel my spirits lift. The vivid landscapes are so huge, so bright and vibrant that I could almost step into them, and they completely envelop me. I could stare at them all day and, in fact, I do sit and gaze at many of them for ages.

When I leave, I feel as revitalised as if I have been diving into those Californian swimming pools, walking in those East Yorkshire woods. The best thing is that their radiance seems to have imprinted itself onto my retinas, so that when I close my eyes, I can still see them and be transported back to their strength and energy.

So, if you are feeling worn down by the relentless treadmill of illness, my advice would be to go to a gallery. Many of them are free. Stare at fields of sunflowers, pools of waterlilies, squares of red and orange or explosions of paint. They will transport you a million miles from hospital beds, waiting rooms and corridors. Maybe buy some postcards to remind yourself afterwards – I have mine pinned up in my kitchen. And if you want to help a friend, being taken to look at some paintings certainly worked for me.

Healing harmonies

The emotional energy of music can be hugely beneficial to mental health. Many have observed that even when people are held tight in the clutches of dementia or depression, music can loosen its grasp in a way that nothing else can. As Billy Joel once said: 'I think music in itself is healing. It's an explosive expression of humanity.' Alan never lost his ability to enjoy listening to his favourite music and now attends a brilliant monthly music-therapy session. Everyone in the group nominates a favourite song on a specific theme, the music is played via YouTube on a large screen and the group then chats about the memories the music evokes. Simple, but highly effective.

I found that classical music, particularly Mozart and Bach, never failed to soothe and comfort. I found that upbeat happy pop songs could lift me on a hard day but sometimes they grated. I found that it could be cathartic to listen to sad music and cry, and that *Fix You* by Coldplay, *Human* by The Killers and *Bridge over Troubled Water* by Simon & Garfunkel helped me.

The intensity of the wrong song at the wrong time can be overwhelming. I was driving back from the hospital late one evening, and the track *Brain Damage* from Pink Floyd's 1973 album *The Dark Side of the Moon* came on the radio. The lines about the 'lunatic in my head', which are accompanied by manic laughter, were way too much and I had to pull over (not easy on a three-lane roundabout) to calm down. But I have since found out that this same song has actually helped people who are struggling with mental health issues; you just have to find the music that works for you.

Ten pieces of instrumental classical music to soothe your soul

- *Prelude No 1* (BWV 846) by Bach
- *Serenade in G Major* (*Eine Kleine Nachtmusik K525*), second movement, by Mozart
- *The Swan* (from the *Carnival of the Animals*) by Saint-Saëns
- *Largo* from *Serse* (HWV 40) by Handel
- *Nocturne* (Opus 9, No 2) by Chopin
- *Moonlight Sonata* (Opus 27, No 2), first movement, by Beethoven
- *Canon in D* by Pachelbel
- *Air on the G String*, Wilhelmj's arrangement of the second movement of Bach's *Orchestral Suite No 3*
- *The Lark Ascending* by Vaughan Williams
- *Largo* from *Winter: The Four Seasons* (*Violin Concerto No 4*) by Vivaldi

Just an old sweet song

A year before Alan himself was ill, his 94-year-old father, beloved 'Grandpa Spode', was in a different hospital, at the end of a life well lived. He had been moved into his own room, and Alan was just about to drive down to Croydon to see him, when I had an idea. He loved music, and we had enjoyed many an evening listening to old jazz standards together. I suggested Alan took with him a small speaker and my iPod with a playlist of the gentle nostalgic tunes I knew were Grandpa's favourites. Al said afterwards that as soon as he pressed play, the atmosphere in the room changed. Even though Grandpa could no longer talk, I'm certain he could still hear. He died a few days later, and it was a great comfort to us to think that on that final evening he drifted away to the familiar music of Irving Berlin, Fats Waller, Ray Noble, George Gershwin and Glen Miller. If you have a relative in hospital, I highly recommend playing music to them that you know they love, through headphones if necessary. Study after study has shown that music reaches parts of the brain that other things don't, and its calming qualities are well attested to.

I love you just the way you are

Nowadays with Alan, I am sometimes struck by the similarities between caring for him and working with children with autism, during my six years as a learning support assistant in a primary school. There are many things he can do perfectly, but there are many that are beyond him. There is the same inability to see a situation through someone else's eyes, the same requirement for simple 'one step' explanations. And much of the time, as with autism, it isn't obvious to other people that he's not 'seeing' things the way they are. On occasions, Alan is adamant that something has happened recently even though it hasn't. He will say, 'I know you say this is true, and I know you aren't lying. But I can't believe it. I know I have to believe it, but I can't.' And I am reminded of the training I had to enable me to work with autistic children, when I needed to fully understand how very differently they perceived the world in order to help them.

It is intensely frustrating, but sometimes it is easier for us to try and appreciate how Alan thinks than it is to convince him that he is wrong and we are right. And the thing that is hardest of all is that he doesn't really understand how profoundly different he is to the Alan he used to be.

I am also sometimes reminded of my wonderful cousin Jane, who has Down's Syndrome, and aged 52 is living a full, rewarding life. To everyone in the family, she has always been a complex, funny, determined human being; both perfect and imperfect like the rest of us. We know there are limits to what she can and can't do, and so does she, although like any other person, she is always exploring her own boundaries. Does Jane know that she moves through the world differently to 99% of other people? I don't know.

I was struck years ago by an article in a parenting magazine about what it was like to have a baby with Down's. The mother likened it to thinking you were going to Italy on holiday. You were looking forward to the culture, the scenery, the food, the architecture, the weather. Then the plane lands in the Netherlands. Of course, Holland is great, but you are going to have to make a major adjustment to your expectations. The issue I have is that we have landed in Holland, but Alan still thinks he's in Italy.

Alan's therapists quite often said to me that their job was

to 'get Alan back'. It's a well-meaning objective but deeply misleading. On a difficult day, it can be as annoying a remark as suggesting your child could be cured of their autism or hypothesising what they might be like if they weren't in a wheelchair. Deep down, of course, Alan is the same person as he was pre brain injury. But on many levels, he isn't. And for us as a family, I believe that adapting to and accepting the new Alan is much more important than forever searching for the old one.

Chapter Twelve

USING THE OUTSIDE TO HELP THE INSIDE

The Healing Power of Nature

Nature's balm

During Alan's long stay on the hospital's neurology ward, he couldn't leave the building for the first three months, but finally in early April, the doctors decide he is well enough to go outside. I have been desperate for this moment and believe that for Al to feel the sun on his face, and hear the sound of birds and the rustling of trees, must be a good thing. The large building faces one of the busiest and most traffic-clogged roads in the entire city, and the outside space consists of an unprepossessing mess of 1970s concrete, some grubby sculptures, a taxi rank, lots of smokers and a grimy pond.

But then I find a wonderful, slightly secret little oasis built by a charity. There are warm wooden benches, leafy shrubs and silver birch trees set against vibrant walls, which shield us from the buses and cars. To begin with, it is easier to push him in a wheelchair, as the long months in bed have meant that he often falls. Accompanied by a nurse, we sit and appreciate the warm spring air. Truthfully, it is as beneficial for me as it is for him; the clinical claustrophobia of the hospital air has been intense. From then on, we try and go outside as often as possible.

From June, once Alan is staying in the Brain Rehab Centre, we get into the habit of going into the garden as soon as we arrive; it is infinitely nicer than his small, dark room. There are trees and flowers, but despite the fact that they are in full bloom, and Alan is in shorts and a T-shirt, he will still frequently suggest that it is winter and maybe too cold to be outside. Eventually, we are allowed to take him for walks to a nearby park. It is beautiful, and again I talk about the trees, the enormous sky, the views across the city. But Alan is so closed in on himself that it is a constant effort to get him to look outward rather than inward. One afternoon in August, we are sitting on the heath with a heat haze rising from the grass, the trees gently rustling and birds chirruping, and he comments that it will soon be Christmas. His poor brain is often so focused on when it can next switch off, sleep and recharge that there seems to be no energy left to notice anything else. But we persevere, and slowly, slowly he becomes more aware of his surroundings. He comes home, and we walk round parks, down streets, along the river and I say, 'Look at the flowers, look at the trees, isn't this nice?' 'Lovely,' he always replies automatically.

And then, one November day, almost two years after he has come out of hospital, we are sweeping up leaves outside our house. Suddenly I notice that he is standing stock-still, staring. I am concerned, maybe he is too tired and needs to sit down – this happens sometimes, he abruptly runs out of oomph. But he is transfixed by the sight of our neighbour's tree, a 50-foot gingko, its bright leaves like thousands of golden coins thrown into the blue sky. 'Look at that tree,' he marvels. 'Just look at that tree, isn't it wonderful?' This is the first time he has initiated a comment on the beauty of the world we live in, and I silently rejoice.

A room with a view

In 1984, researcher and author Professor Roger S. Ulrich published some ground-breaking research which showed that a natural view may help patients recover faster after surgery. Between 1974 and 1981, he compared patients recovering from surgery in a hospital in Pennsylvania, who had a window in their room that looked out onto a view of leafy trees, with others whose windows looked onto a brick wall. The patients were carefully evaluated and 'matched' so that, as far as possible, all other conditions were similar. He found that those with a view had shorter hospital stays, received fewer negative evaluative comments in nurses' notes and took fewer strong painkillers.

This study examining the restorative effect of natural views has now gone on to influence hospital design worldwide, including the size and location of windows in wards. Ulrich believes that 'because most natural views apparently foster positive feelings, reduce fear in stressed subjects, hold interest and may block or reduce stressful thoughts, they might also foster restoration from anxiety or stress'. Other studies have also shown that views of nature can have important benefits in terms of improving clinical outcomes. One study in Sweden (1993), for example, investigated whether exposing heart surgery patients to pictures of nature would improve recovery. In total, 160 patients in intensive care were given simulated views of either trees and water, abstract pictures, a white panel or no picture. Results suggested that patients who viewed the trees and water scene were significantly less anxious during the postoperative period and suffered less severe pain, as evidenced by the fact that they moved more quickly than the other groups from strong narcotic pain drugs onto something more moderate.

Ulrich has also presented research (2002) into the importance of having gardens in hospitals, suggesting that they 'will likely calm or ameliorate stress effectively if they contain verdant foliage, flowers, water or harmonious nature sounds and visible wildlife'. His research shows that both 'laboratory and clinical investigations have found that viewing nature settings can produce significant restoration within less than five minutes as indicated by positive changes, for instance, in blood pressure, heart activity, muscle tension, and brain electrical activity'. The belief that plants and gardens are beneficial for patients in healthcare environments is, of course, thousands of years old, and both the early hospitals and monasteries often had soothing gardens that were used for recovery and meditation, as well as providing medicinal herbs.

Blowing away the dark humours

I hear a palliative care nurse, Rachel Clarke, who has written an inspiring book (*Dear Life: A Doctor's Story of Love and Loss*), talking on the radio about how important nature often is for people at the end of their lives. She speaks about one breast cancer patient, who loved the natural world and got a great deal of comfort from being outside. 'She found a kind of peace in accepting that her cycle, her life cycle had a natural beginning and end as well.' Rachel went on to say that even though patients are often believed to be too unwell to leave the hospice, she is a great believer in wheeling their beds into the garden. She recalls how often patients have 'an almost beatific smile on their face as they're feeling that winter sunshine, listening to the birds and the trees'.

Filmmaker Derek Jarman, when he was diagnosed as HIV positive in 1986 (at that time, a death sentence), opted to plant a garden in the stony shingle around his home by the beach in Dungeness. He wrote in his journals of the pleasure he found in it. 'Crystalline sunlight. All the dark humours blown away by the wind. The crocuses open quickly, bright yellow petals spread open by noon. The purple and white in the shadows.'

Playwright Dennis Potter spoke emotively in an interview on Channel 4, right at the end of his life, when he was dying of pancreatic cancer, of the intense power and beauty of the natural world. He recalled gazing at a flowering plum tree, and rather than just thinking how nice it looked, he saw that it was 'the whitest, frothiest, blossomest blossom that there ever could be'. The splendour of the tree struck him forcefully, and he described how he felt that 'the nowness of everything is absolutely wondrous'.

The seeds of regrowth

Nowadays, Alan goes to a Day Respite Centre every Tuesday and I have five hours to myself, which I largely spend walking. I don't quite know where the decision to do this came from, but when I first began the habit, as soon as I walked into the forest of ancient trees in the large park near my home, I could feel tears running down my face and something heavy lifting from my shoulders. There is something about the age and permanence of the mighty oaks and chestnuts that is enormously soothing. They seem to be saying, 'We understand. We are here and we will still be here when your troubles are not. This will pass. We are old and we have seen it all before.'

Maybe trees can sense how you feel. I'm certainly not the only person to feel this. Judi Dench thinks of the trees in her garden as part of her 'extended family', and believes 'there is much more to these magical giants' than we realise, in how they 'live, breathe and communicate'. German forester Peter Wohlleben, in his wonderful book *The Hidden Life of Trees: What They Feel, How They Communicate: Discoveries from a Secret World*, comes up with many examples and explanations of how and why trees interact with their environment, finding that 'every day in the forest was a day of discovery' and that 'perhaps we are poorer for having lost a possible explanation or richer for having gained a mystery'.

Every week I walk in the woods, and seeing the same trees, slightly changed every time, is powerfully healing. They are still but they are also constantly moving; put your ear to the trunk and you can almost hear them growing, as well as the scuffle and stir of insects and birds living in them. They are both passive and active. They can listen but not answer. I don't know why, but I can say for certain that walking among trees makes me feel better.

Shinrin-yoku (forest bathing)

Shinrin-yoku is a nature therapy originating in Japan that research has proven to have health benefits. It was developed in the 1980s and is now an important part of Japanese preventative healthcare. It's a simple idea: if you visit a wood and walk round it in a relaxed manner, you will become rejuvenated, revitalised and restored. There's lots of research to back up this idea. For example, one study (2014) showed that subjects who took a leisurely forest walk, compared with an urban walk, showed a 12.4% decrease in the stress hormone cortisol, a 1.4% decrease in blood pressure and a 5.8% decrease in heart rate. Another (2008) found that the chemicals secreted by evergreen trees (known as phytoncide) were associated with improvements in the functioning of the patients' immune systems. And another (2010) found that men taking two-hour walks in the woods over a two-day period exhibited a 50% increase in levels of 'antiviral cells', which the body uses to fight disease.

The idea isn't new. In the 1800s, physicians Peter Dettweiler and Hermann Brehmer set up sanatoriums for treating tuberculosis in Germany's pine forests, as did Edward Trudeau in the Adirondack forests of New York. They found that the health of their patients improved because of their surroundings, referred to as the 'forest cure', and speculated that perhaps the pine trees were secreting a healing balm into the air.

I read a really interesting study (2015) entitled 'The Benefits of Group Walking in Forests for People with Significant Mental Ill-Health' and based on a pilot programme in Ireland, 'Woodland for Health', which investigated the effects of group walking in forests for people with significant mental ill health, including depression, bipolar and anxiety disorders. It finds that 'individuals with major depressive disorders experienced improved moods immediately after nature walks' and that 'nature could be a regarded as a "co-therapist" for healing mental ill-health'.

Green prescriptions

The more I look into it, the more I see that this idea is catching on everywhere. In Shetland, doctors are already issuing 'green prescriptions'. Karen MacKelvie, a community engagement officer, organised some research on the benefits of connecting people with nature in a bid to overcome growing mental health problems and the causes behind many long-term conditions. 'Nature prescribing' became reality after a successful pilot project, and all GP surgeries across the islands now have a leaflet explaining the potential benefits of interaction with nature: reduction of hypertension; reduced respiratory tract and cardiovascular problems and anxiety; improved concentration and mood; even increased life satisfaction and happiness. GPs have different lengths of walks to prescribe, as well as suggestions for activities to connect with nature. The evidence base for similar schemes is growing. A project in England from the Centre for Sustainable Healthcare, called Prescribing Green Space, found 'that six to eight months after receiving a "green prescription" – where people are encouraged to help plant forests and spend time in local green spaces – 63% of patients were more active and 46% had lost weight'.

Rachel Halliwell, a journalist, credits her doctor's advice with her return to more robust mental and physical health. 'Get a pot, put some soil and a seed in it, stick it on a windowsill and nurture the plant that grows,' said her GP, rather than giving her pills. 'And next time you feel like sliding down the nearest wall, go for a walk.'

Dr Arun Ghosh, a GP in Liverpool, says that:

modern human beings are disconnected from nature for too much of the time and we're paying the price with our mental health. We're meant to be outdoors, breathing fresh air, not stuck inside with the phone constantly ringing and rarely feeling the sun on our heads. Just looking after a plant – which will always grow at its own pace – gets you engaged in a simple process with a natural cycle that reminds you exactly where you come from as a human being.

Walk yourself well

The early months of visiting Alan mostly involve moving through a very urban environment to a very clinical one, and the lack of green space has a bad effect on my mood. Then a friend, who has also had a relation in the hospital for a long time, gives me a fabulous tip. She advises me to stay on the train for one more stop. This means that the walk will no longer involve a 15-minute stride down a busy pavement, alongside a road clogged with buses, cars and ambulances, but instead will take me through a cemetery. This is a tranquil space, full of trees that, at the point when I discover it, are just coming into leaf. Hundred-year-old gravestones nestle in long grass; there are blackbirds, blue tits and cheeky squirrels. On the mornings when I am full of trepidation as to what the day will bring, the walk through the cemetery calms me. And in the afternoons when I leave, sometimes full of misery, the peaceful surroundings soothe me. When I close my eyes at night, the recollection of the bright daffodils or the budding trees replaces the fluorescent lighting and sterile corridors that are imprinted on my retinas.

Nowadays, ensuring that Alan and I try to have a walk every day to look at something green, even if it is just the neighbours' front gardens or the grass in the small park over the road, is important for both of us. Alan doesn't usually remember that he's been on a walk, but I am certain that its benefits are lodged somewhere in his brain.

All creatures great and small

I sit in my garden one early evening in high summer. I've just got back from the long trek of walk-bus-train-train required to visit the Brain Rehab Centre. There was a difficult conversation with Alan's therapists about his lack of motivation, then the trains were playing silly buggers and, after all that coupled with rush hour, I'm feeling frazzled. I'm watching a trail of ants march out of a small hole in the wall, gather up tiny bits of leaf and then head back into the bricks, via a different route. They are well organised; some are in charge of collection, others seem to be walking for no apparent reason, but maybe they're protecting the others. They all look purposeful. I think how odd it is that I am watching them so closely, and yet I know nothing of their world, their challenges or triumphs. I think of Robert the Bruce, a medieval king of Scotland, who sat in a cave watching a spider spin and respin a web and realised that perseverance and persistence were what was needed in his own life.

Sitting and watching the ants, birds or bees seems to make me feel better. I think it is partly a question of scale; the fluid, deliberate movement of thousands of tiny creatures makes you realise that you may be bigger, but you are not necessarily more important. And watching the natural world go about its business is a healthy reminder that your world is not the only one. Yours is not the only galaxy in the universe; you are not the only cog in the wheel.

The circle of life

One of the cruellest things about Alan's lack of working memory is that it means it is almost impossible for him to measure his own recovery. The passing of the months or years – or even the advancement of just one day – is often meaningless to him. But for me, as I look after him, getting some sense of progress, of change and of growth is essential, and I've found there is nothing better at helping with this than nature. Getting out into the garden and pruning a rose or planting a bulb is an affirmation that you can envisage a future, a brighter time ahead. And the most encouraging thing of all is that even when you don't do anything at all to help it, nature will renew itself.

The winter when Alan is first ill, I am in the hospital all day and hardly get out into the garden, but it's still all there, quietly sprouting and swelling. In early spring, Alice comes and sweeps away all the leaves and winter debris, and Ginny helps me prune back our rampant rambling rose. Seeing new shoots springing up everywhere is incredibly invigorating. My garden is pushing itself back to life just as Alan's body is trying to do.

Gardener Monty Don has spoken movingly about the positive effects of gardening on health. 'That first snowdrop, the flowering of the rose you pruned, a lettuce you grew from seed, the robin singing just for you. These are small things but all positive, all healing in a way that medicine tries to mimic.' And nowadays, even if Alan can't remember doing any gardening, showing him that something he has done has reaped rewards, even if it's just raking leaves or mowing the lawn, is a good way to bring structure into his muddled brain. As Monty Don says:

Gardening is a good way to find beauty in chaos. By becoming in tune with the seasons of growth and fall, preparation and harvest you make your mind and body happier and healthier. By having a direct stake and involvement with the process of plants growing, of having your hands in the soil and tending it carefully and with love, your world, and everyone else's world too, becomes a better place.

How nature can help you

- Have a ten-minute walk every single day, whatever the weather.
- Plant something. A sunflower seed, a bulb, a conker. You will see progress.
- When you are out and about, take a close-up photo on your phone of something natural. Look at its detail and marvel. Enjoy focusing on something other than yourself.
- Bring something natural indoors, just a sprig of greenery in a glass of water will do.
- Sit outside with a cup of tea. Listen to the air.
- Stand with bare feet on the grass.
- Watch birds, bees, butterflies, ants. They will give you the sense that your world is not the only one that matters.
- Look at, listen to, touch – and yes, even hug – a tree.

Chapter Thirteen

RECOVERY

Normal Service will not be Resumed

Managing expectations

WHAT IS RECOVERY? THERE'S an old joke about an Irishman, who is asked by a motorist who has gone off course how he can get to his destination. The Irishman stands and thinks for a long time before eventually saying, 'Well, I wouldn't start from here.' That's how recovery feels. Your initial instinct is to remember the point at which the patient was perfectly well, and then hope against hope that they will eventually get back to being that person again. But where you need to measure from is the moment when the patient was at their most ill. Recovery is not about trying to get back to where you were but moving forward to where you are going.

Everyone likes a happy ending, and friends can be shocked when the answer to 'So, do you feel you've got the old Alan back then?' is 'No.' The children and I found it infuriating, but also funny, how many people immediately linked the fact that he was coming home in late November with the imminent arrival of the festive season. 'Ahh, how fantastic that he's home for Christmas,' friends cried, as if he was being transported by Santa himself, and the truth that he'd been in hospital for the whole year, missing birthdays, anniversaries, graduation ceremonies and holidays, was swept away in one joyous Christmas miracle.

The father returning home after a long absence is such a familiar scene in popular culture, from *Little Women* to *The Railway Children* to *Stick Man*, that it seemed almost churlish to deny to well-wishers that there had been a 'Daddy, oh my Daddy' moment. All year we'd been thinking of how joyful we would be when Alan came home, and when the great day finally arrived, we were indeed full of relief and gratitude, but at the same time very aware that the road ahead would be a bumpy one.

However, the Hollywood-style reunion scene was luckily supplied by Lola, our small Havanese. Unlike the rest of us, of course, she had been unable to visit Alan, and for many months he didn't even remember that we had a dog. And we had no way of knowing whether Lola missed him or not; she is a cheery little thing and certainly didn't appear to be moping around the place or pining. But when he walked back through our front door, her utter joy was plain to see. She made a funny little squeaking noise, which we'd never heard before, and literally bounced non-stop with happiness, springing round and round Alan as if she couldn't quite believe her eyes. At the same time, she clearly knew he was ill, and when she snuggled up to him on the sofa, she licked and nudged him very, very gently, most unlike her usual boisterous self.

'You must be so happy he's home!'

The discrepancy between recovery for the patient and recovery for the carer is a taboo subject. Of course, I was overjoyed to have Alan home, but in many ways, it almost immediately made my life harder and more complicated. I no longer had to make the long drive or train journey to visit him, but from now on, my time was not my own – it was always shared. For almost a year, I had been able to plan out my time to suit myself; now every moment had to be arranged around Alan. He couldn't be alone, and when I was with him, I had to always be thinking about what he was doing, or going to do, next. I thought my day would be full of worry about whether he might start having seizures again or fall down the stairs, or whether I'd remember to give him the right pills at the right time, but in fact it was much more mundane than that. I spent hours saying the same things again and again, making schedules, reassuring him, explaining. It was a relief when he had a nap, and then I'd feel guilty for thinking that.

A nice OT came round to help him settle in and rather coyly suggested we go out on 'date nights'. I smiled politely but inside I was seething in horror. I was already spending 24 hours a day looking after Alan – quite literally, since he often woke in the night; what I looked forward to was time by myself or with other people. I certainly wasn't about to start organising intimate dinners for two. I remembered the tired woman I had met in hospital with the grumpy husband, who didn't want him to come home and whose life ahead looked like it was going to be pretty rubbish. Hugh Marriott, in his excellent book *The Selfish Pig's Guide to Caring*, says, 'What goes on in the minds and deep despairing souls of the carers is a complete unknown. Except to other carers. They know. They've been there.'

Adjusting and adapting

It can't be overestimated how long it might take the patient to adjust to a new situation. For us, the situation was complicated by the fact that Alan couldn't remember any of his time in hospital or the Brain Rehab Centre. In his mind, he felt as if just a few days earlier he had been at work, driving his car and running his business, as if the whole of 2017 hadn't happened. You might think this was a good thing, but of course it brought a whole different set of problems. But for many patients, getting used to the difference between being in hospital, where many highly skilled professionals are focused on helping you, and a home environment, where you just have to 'get on with it', can be acute and very difficult.

There can also be a huge discrepancy between the feelings of a family who are thankful for what they've gained and a patient who is mourning what they've lost. For me, it was, and still is, a delicate balancing act. If I remind Alan that he isn't working, driving or living anything resembling an independent life, then he is sad. In the early days, he was more than sad, he was devastated. But if I didn't remind him of these things, he was permanently stuck in the land of make-believe and it was impossible for him to live his new life in any meaningful way. With dementia, I know that it is often kinder to allow a patient to live in their own bubble of delusion. But Alan's brain injury is not degenerative, so it is possible for him to adapt and move forward.

However, it has taken many years of repetition for him to even begin to grasp the enormity of what has happened to him. He no longer gazes endlessly up and down the street looking for his car or insists that he needs to do some work on his laptop ready for an appointment tomorrow. On one level, he has learnt new habits and adapted to a different way of life. But he is still a lot happier if he doesn't look backward, forward or inward, and for him, 'coming to terms' with what has happened is still very much a work in progress.

Journalist Simon Hattenstone, who had encephalitis as a child, writes that he divided his 'life into BE and AE, before encephalitis and after encephalitis. Not simply because it was significant for me, but because I had emerged from the illness a different person.' Some patients recover enough to be able to perceive this difference in themselves, and sadly some do not. Alan falls into the latter category.

Sometimes people say to us, 'Oh, he seems just the same to me,' and I think, 'Yes, but that's because you are only seeing the "public" Alan.' It's true, he's largely regained his ability to chat to absolutely anyone, to laugh and make jokes, to fit in. But the husband I had – the one who empathised, sympathised, encouraged, hypothesised, planned, reflected and conjectured, who *understood* – he's gone. I'll never lose the grief of this, but I believe I can learn to live with it.

The long and winding road

One of the hardest things to cope with is the concept that although a patient may be 'better' when they come home, 'better' doesn't always mean 'completely better' and they may be left with serious after-effects that will need a lot of time to adjust to. The lasting effects can be physical or mental or both, and whether it's learning to live with extreme tiredness, a permanent disability, tricky medical equipment or a change in personality, don't underestimate how many months or even years it might take before you begin to feel that you are coping well.

Many ongoing issues are common to specific illnesses, and this is when the charities and societies can be hugely helpful. I found that one of the best things that the Encephalitis Society provided was the reassurance that we were not the only family going through this. One of the things that is hard to comprehend for anyone affected by a brain injury is that the process of 'learning to live with a disability' is fraught with problems, as most 'learning' requires accurate memory! The Encephalitis Society website tells me that 'unfortunately, many people affected by encephalitis do not learn from mistakes but rather learn to repeat those mistakes and explain them away', and I find it very reassuring to see this in black and white on the days when Alan's confabulations are driving me nuts. Neuropsychologist Dr Audrey Daisley says that a common issue for couples following encephalitis is that the partner of the patient is 'particularly vulnerable to the unique loss of "us"', and again, it helps a lot to see this written down.

Rehabilitation, recuperation and restoration

What does rehabilitation mean? When Alan moved from the hospital to the Brain Rehab Centre, it just felt as if he had moved from one hospital environment to another. But in practical terms, the hospital was trying to mend him, whereas the Brain Rehab Centre was trying to help him cope with being broken. And when he came home at the end of 2017, it was really the start of another much longer, ongoing period of rehabilitation. I found this explanation from the Encephalitis Society's website helpful.

Rehabilitation can't...

- return the person to the way they were before
- 'cure' intellectual problems
- help the person cope with any demand placed on them
- take away the distress and heartache caused by the injury.

Rehabilitation can...

- provide coping skills and greater independence in everyday life
- help reintegration into the community and family life
- improve emotional adjustment
- develop social skills and re-integration
- help and support families to cope
- improve the quality of life.

The importance of routine

Aside from the twee suggestions about date nights, the OT who comes to our house has lots of good practical advice about how we can help Alan adjust to being at home. By far the most useful suggestion is to stress the importance of routine for someone with a brain injury. They help me to construct a daily timetable, which we stick up on the kitchen wall. Every hour of the day is blocked in with very simple things like '9am–10am read papers' and '11am–12pm snooze' and '4–5pm tea and chat with family'. Initially, I didn't really understand how vital this structure was for someone with any sort of brain injury. But now I can see that 'the schedule' has been a major contributor to Alan's recovery; in fact, I think it is the single most important factor. For someone whose mind is jumbled, this creation of form, a rationale to the days, is vital.

Over the months, Alan gets more and more used to the idea that there is a plan to his life. Very gradually, he stops aimlessly wandering, stops feeling that there is something else he's meant to be doing and stops worrying about nebulous concepts.

People ask me all the time whether Alan is getting better. And it's a question that is very hard to answer – because he *is* getting better – but not in the way that they probably mean. The single biggest improvement has been that he now accepts that there is a pattern to his life that he has no control over. He knows that if he wants to know what is happening then he will need to ask me or look at something written down. And he is now unquestioning and accepting of this. And in fact, by sticking to a routine most of the time, when we do step outside it and do something new or different, he is much more able to cope, as if his brain is comforted by the knowledge that this is only temporary and normal service will soon be resumed.

Every morning, I wake Alan up at 9am. 'What am I doing today?' he asks. As he does every day. When I tell him it's an entirely unremarkable day with allocated times for reading the paper, meals, watching TV, chatting with the family, walking and naps, he is pleased. 'Excellent, a really good day then,' he says. Much of my role as his carer is to prompt, to remind, to organise, to help. There are things he couldn't possibly do for himself, like organising his medication or going somewhere else; there are things he can do with help, like finding his clothes. There are thousands of us around the country having very similar days while looking after our partners, and I know some are dealing with much more difficult physical labour than I am – pushing wheelchairs, endlessly washing sheets, administering injections, etc. But I suspect many carers would agree that the three hardest things are:

- the unrelenting 'sameyness' of it all

- adapting to the change from the existence you both used to have

- trying to fit in having a life of your own around being entirely responsible for someone else's.

It's OK to be angry

One summer lunchtime, six months or so after Alan has come home, we are driving into the countryside for lunch with friends. In the past, Alan has usually done most of the driving and I've done the navigating; that's been our style for 30 years, and it's suited us, up and down the UK and France, using fat spiral-bound Michelin maps and then more recently a satnav. Sure, we've had the odd argument – the family can all recall an incident with the autoroute junctions around Rouen – but we've been a good team. We've found remote holiday houses even when the instructions have been unintelligible, we've discovered the perfect picnic places down the unlikeliest of roads. And Alan was the sort of driver who seemed to instinctively know which way was the right way and who'd always remember if he'd been somewhere before.

But nowadays, aside from his general lack of memory, something has gone permanently askew in the location-finding part of his brain. He can't always find his way around his own house, and he certainly can't read a map. So, I'm doing both the driving and the navigation, and it's not going well. Deep into the Hampshire countryside, we're hopelessly lost, there's no mobile phone signal and we've just passed a farm gate that we've already driven past twice. 'Well, we've definitely never been down this road before,' Al remarks helpfully. It's hot, we're late and I totally lose my temper. The frustration comes pouring out and I shout and rail for about five minutes, although I know it's not his fault and it's really unkind. And the worst thing is that Alan just sits there quietly. He doesn't argue back, and this passivity is one of the things I find the hardest to deal with; it's just so unlike the old Alan.

The other thing that is strangely frightening is that I know Alan won't remember this. It's not like a normal row, where you might grump for a bit or laugh about it afterwards. Whatever I say now, Alan won't remember. This is scary; it feels as if there are no limitations on my temper, and dark thoughts crowd into my head of the carers you read about who snap under pressure. I sit in silence for a while, then pull myself together, have another look at the instructions and work out where we've gone wrong. Sure enough, when we arrive and my friend asks if we found her house alright, Alan blithely assures her, with no hint of irony or deception, that it has been a really easy drive. He simply doesn't remember my meltdown.

As time goes by

Measuring recovery is difficult. In hospital, there is a young woman in the room next to Alan's who lies in bed for weeks, seemingly comatose. She has no visitors. We thank our lucky stars that Alan is not as ill as she is. Over the months, she gradually starts to sit up and then move around. She starts to wander, sometimes trying to grab other patients, drifting into their rooms. She never speaks and it's hard not to be slightly frightened by her. One day I notice that Alan's fingernails are really long and ask a nurse if she has some nail scissors. To both of our amusement, she tells me that despite the armoury of potions, pills and all manner of medical implements she has in her possession, scissors are not a regulation NHS-issued item. Suddenly, the young woman from next door appears in the room, and I'm unnerved by her abrupt and silent presence. But she puts out her hand, looking at me and then Alan, and in it are a small pair of nail scissors. I thank her, as I realise that many of my assumptions about her mental abilities are wrong. In the coming weeks, she improves still further, and of course we are pleased for her, but privately, we all agree that it's hard not to feel disheartened that she is getting better so much faster than Alan is.

On our first full day at the Brain Rehab Centre, a nurse makes Alan and me a mug of tea along with one for another man, who is sitting at the communal kitchen table. I take ours out into the garden, and she places the other man's mug in front of him. Out of the corner of my eye, I see him moving his hand, very slowly, towards the mug. When I come back ten minutes later in search of biscuits, his hand has only just reached the handle. I glance at the nurse, wondering why she isn't helping him, and then I realise that, of course, he must do it himself. Painstakingly, laboriously, he starts to raise the mug to his lips. Half an hour later we come inside, and the hand with the mug in still hasn't reached his mouth. By now, the tea in it is obviously stone cold. By the time we leave the Brain Rehab Centre, six months later, the man is walking to the kettle and making his own tea, as well as drinking it with ease.

In the early days of Alan's recovery in hospital, we decide that playing patience will be a good, mindful activity for him. He's often played it at home as a relaxation tool after a day at work. Watching him trying to do it now is a sobering illustration of the scrambled chaos inside his head. It reminds me of photos I have seen of what happens if you give a spider a tiny injection of caffeine – the web it spins is crazily haphazard, and the way Alan tries to arrange the cards is equally random. Over the years, he has gradually relearnt it: the order of the numbers, what goes where, how to progress, when it's over. Nowadays he can lay out the cards on our breakfast bar without difficulty.

The point of these three anecdotes is to illustrate that sometimes the tangible signs of recovery can show you what is happening inside someone's head and sometimes they can't. But without physical indications, it's difficult to measure progress. My friend Maria gave me a bracelet for my 50th birthday, before Alan was ill, with the engraved inscription 'Don't look back, you're not going that way', but I think sometimes you *do* need to look back, in order to see how far you've come.

Relapse

Five months after Alan has come home, there is a sudden and dramatic change. He has a normal day, but then at about 2am he gets out of bed and starts wandering around looking for sausages. I persuade him to get back into bed and go back to sleep, but then 25 minutes later it happens again, And again and again – all night long. Every time the reason for getting up is different. Sometimes he needs to go to work, sometimes he has to sort out the baby, sometimes he has to cook supper. He has no idea where he is and is extremely agitated. The next morning, he can't remember anything about it. I wonder if it is perhaps a slight infection or a tummy bug; these things have thrown him off course before. But the next night it happens again. It is horribly frightening, and apart from this, being woken up every 15 minutes takes its toll on me, and I feel as if I am going completely crazy myself.

The next morning, I email his neurology consultant, who gets back to me immediately and tells me to bring him straight in. Although they are expecting us, the point of entry is, nevertheless, via A&E. Alan is utterly exhausted and does not understand what is happening. We wait in a narrow corridor for a long, long time. Alan has a chair; at some point I give mine to a woman who is clearly in a lot of pain with stomach cramps. And we wait.

My year of hospitals has armed me with a certain degree of both stoicism and preparation. I have the most important things: a phone, a charger, books, water. But I cannot do anything to help Alan who gets more and more agitated. He alternates between falling asleep and wanting to walk around and leave; every time he gets up, I have to stop other people taking his chair. It is horrendous, and my own tiredness contributes to the claustrophobia of the situation. I start to feel that we will never be seen, that we will be trapped here forever.

Eventually, after several hours, I need to go to the loo. The woman next to me, who has of course heard all of our increasingly fraught conversations, kindly says she'll keep an eye on him, and I dash off. When I return, five minutes later, both Alan and the woman are gone. I can't believe it at first: there are now completely different patients sitting on the chairs, and it is as if Alan has never been here. I burst into tears and frantically find a nurse. She looks at me as if I am hugely overreacting, and says, 'Well, he's obviously in with one of the doctors, I'm sure he'll be out in a minute.' When I explain to her that he doesn't know where he is and could easily have just decided to leave the building to look for me, she sighs, 'He could be in any of the consulting rooms.' We look together at all the closed white doors. 'And, there's no way of knowing which doctor called him,' she says. By now I am at breaking point. 'Yes, there is,' I say. 'We can knock on each of these doors and see if he's in there.'

She can see I mean it, and reluctantly she begins knocking on each door and asking if Mr Jessop is there. I am frantic with worry that by now he is wandering around on the main road outside, and the relief when a doctor says 'yes' is indescribable. The nurse apologises, but the doctor looks at me with undisguised relief. 'Ah good, Mrs Jessop,' he says. 'I'm glad you're here, I think we need you. Your husband has just been explaining to me about the fertility problems he's been having. Apparently, you've come in to see me because you're trying to have a baby?!?' This time I burst into hysterical laughter, and in a relatively short time, the A&E doctor ascertains that Alan certainly does need to be admitted, and by that evening he is back on the neurology ward. A blood test confirms that the antibodies that shouldn't be in his blood are back, and another dose of Rituximab, the super-strong drug that will get rid of them, is ordered. Within days of having it dripped into him, Alan has returned to 'normal'.

In the months immediately following this relapse, this possibility that Alan will become ill again means that every time he is slightly 'off', Sam and I go into a state of red alert. We frequently compare worried notes after Alan has gone to bed: 'Did you notice...?' 'Did you hear...?' 'Does he seem...?' But gradually, we come to notice that being extremely tired or in an unfamiliar place can also cause his brain to go utterly haywire, but a long sleep tends to result in a 'reboot'.

And eventually, the relapse, although truly horrendous, actually has a positive effect. Seeing that Alan could get ill again means that the fear of this occurring is now not as huge. The known is better than the unknown. Yes, I do worry that it might happen again, but the fact that we have coped, and that the hospital and Alan's neurologist are both close, is reassuring. And I realise that living in a constant state of anxiety about things that may or may not happen is not feasible.

The new normal

About a year after his relapse, and on a Tuesday when Alan goes to a Day Respite Centre, I am sitting on the grass, having a solitary picnic in the lovely rose garden that I frequently walk in. There must be over a hundred rose bushes here, all of them glorious, from crimson, cerise and fuchsia through to soft pale pinks and purest white. The smell is utterly intoxicating. A low murmur of bees mingles with the distant shrieks of children on a school trip who are supposed to be observing nature, but instead are daring each other to run under the watering sprays. I realise that I feel... content. Happy.

Just then, a woman walks past me, and we smile at each other. Then she makes a little grimace of annoyance. 'It would be just so lovely if it weren't for the aeroplanes, wouldn't it?' she says. The garden is close to an airport, and it is true; every so often a jet roars overhead. I have genuinely grown so used to the sound that it doesn't disturb me, but of course she is correct, it is definitely there. In fact, as soon as she mentions it, it seems to get much louder and the buzzing of the bees and laughter of the children fades.

It occurs to me that the background noise of these planes is like living with illness. The nagging worry, the possibility that the encephalitis will come back, the forthcoming scans, the appointment next week to get some test results. It's always there, and it's always going to be there, and sometimes it's horribly intrusive. But, genuinely, I think it will be perfectly possible for us to live our lives smelling the roses and listening to the bees without being constantly aware of the aeroplanes.

You have a choice

I hear an amazing woman called Lisa, talking on BBC Radio Gloucestershire. She was diagnosed with stage-three breast cancer and had chemotherapy. Some years afterwards, to her great surprise (since she'd been told the chemo had destroyed her eggs), she fell pregnant. But then, two weeks before her son was born, she found a lump, had it tested and discovered the cancer had come back. Naturally, this was 'highly emotional', and her first reaction was disbelief. Worse is to come: after she has had a healthy baby boy, a PET scan reveals that the cancer has spread to her sternum bone and chest lymph nodes, and she is now classed as incurable. She recalls how she was 'absolutely destroyed inside, that day broke me. I just couldn't believe that I was given this little miracle and then I might not see him grow up.' But although Lisa couldn't change what had happened, she decided that she could change the way she felt about it. She has always loved fashion, and has resolved that she is going to wear her best clothes and nice make-up every day; she describes it as 'fighting cancer with fashion'. She says that she has come to realise she can either 'wallow in my own self-pity and let it ruin the days, months and years I've got', or 'just crack on and choose to live my best life', and this is the choice she's made. Her words make a great impression on me.

Look after yourself

In the early weeks, I have no room in my brain for anything other than thinking about Alan's health and I don't look after myself at all. Every day I spend either travelling or sitting on an uncomfortable chair by Alan's bed. I twist something in my back at one point, an old shoulder problem flairs up, I'm not sleeping properly and, before long, I start to feel absolutely dreadful.

Helped by friends and family, I can see that this is not sustainable and start to take more time for myself – walking more, swimming and doing yoga. I know it's important, both for me and for the kids. With them having effectively lost one parent to look after them, keeping myself in good health is now doubly necessary. I remind myself of this whenever I feel selfish for prioritising my own needs over Alan's. But the fact is, it's hard to look after yourself properly when you are a carer. One survey (2018) found that carers providing more than 50 hours of care per week are twice as likely to report ill health as those not providing care.

A few years into looking after Alan at home, I have a general health check with my GP (unrelated to my being a carer and just because I'm in my mid 50s). Everything is good. I've had a mammogram, which is clear, my cholesterol is good, my urine is clear, my weight is fine, my heartbeat strong, the nurse is ticking boxes and smiling. Then, right at the end, she says, 'OK, we'll just check your blood pressure, and then we're done.' My blood pressure has always been pleasingly low; I'm a regular blood donor, so have it checked fairly often. So, I'm genuinely astonished when she frowns at the machine and says, 'Ooh, hang on, that's a bit worrying.' She finds another machine, but the result is the same: much too high. And it's still too high when I wear a monitor for 12 hours, to eliminate the 'white-coat effect', which can mean some people's blood pressure shoots up from the stress of being in a medical situation.

I am really cross with myself; how can this be? I thought I was doing so well. I don't want to be 'at greater risk of heart disease, kidney disease, dementia and stroke'. I study the list of things that can affect blood pressure, and it dawns on me. I might be walking, swimming and stretching, but I'm not actually doing anything that raises my heart rate – what would be classed as aerobic exercise. The gentle exercise that is good for Alan isn't good enough for me, and the 30 minutes of cycling that I used to do every day to get to and from work has ceased. Being a carer is not actually a very physical activity, at least not in any useful way.

When we filled in the form, the nurse said to me kindly, 'Oh I'm sure you're running around all day looking after your husband,' but in fact, this is a white lie that doesn't really help anyone. The blood-pressure monitor tells the true story. I hear Dr Rangan Chatterjee talking on the radio about his new book, *Feel Better in 5: Your Daily Plan to Feel Great for Life*, and am struck by what he says about fitting in short bursts of movement to your life, which he calls 'health snacks'. He suggests that the best way to do this is to create habits – like brushing your teeth or cleaning your contact lenses – that you learn to do almost automatically. Alan's and my day already has quite the pattern to it, so adding in a few more routine activities would be easy to do. I decide that if I 'attach' ten minutes of vigorous exercise to the times when I tell Alan to go upstairs for his morning and afternoon naps at 11am and 4pm, those 20 minutes a day should be enough to make a significant difference. I can easily run on the spot or do one of Dr Chatterjee's workouts for ten minutes and then get on with something else. I do feel pretty silly at first, but no one is in the house to see me, and soon it does become a habit. Within a couple of months, to my great relief, my blood pressure has plummeted.

When you are a carer, people tell you all the time to 'look after yourself', but it's all too easy to only notice physical changes, such as putting on weight or feeling tired. What is going on invisibly, inside your brain and body, is just as important, and 'look after yourself' is genuinely vital advice. You just might need to look a bit more closely than you think.

Along came coronavirus

And then, in spring 2020, the weirdest thing happened. That peculiar lurch of the seemingly solid foundations on which we stood happened again. Only this time it happened to the entire world. I'm sure I was not the only person to feel a strange connection between what had previously been a very personal experience and the way everyone on the planet was knocked off kilter.

The feeling that 'this can't really be happening' was suddenly experienced by everyone, along with the surreal out-of-body sensation, the suspicion that you were in a film and the hope that you would wake up one day to discover it was all a dream. That time in 2017 when my head was so full of illness that there was no room for normality, accompanied by intense panic and anxiety, was now the norm. How strange to go from a world where hospitals and disease were only for the unlucky few, to a world where it was all everyone talked about. Just as we had done, people realised that they could adapt to 'a new normal' amazingly fast if they had to. Everyone discovered what we had too: that an overload of medical information made you feel much worse, not better. Many people started to conjecture that the crisis would bring about profound change, the 'things will never be the same again' theory that I remembered so well. Society experienced the same 'time bending' phenomenon we had observed when your 'real' life is on hold and the days pass both slowly and quickly. And of course, the coronavirus pandemic showed everyone who didn't already know just how hard everyone in the healthcare system works and at what cost to their own lives.

And, like others who had already travelled down the road of ill health and were therefore vulnerable, we experienced an extra surge of fear. To begin with, the terror that Alan, with his compromised immune system, would catch COVID-19 was so intense that it threatened to tip Izzy, Madeleine, Sam and me into a collective nervous breakdown. This magnified the nagging concerns that were already swirling around in my head. Alan's health must not become the only health that matters to this family. His survival cannot always be at the expense of the mental wellbeing of all those who love him. Whatever life throws at us – even something as terrible as a global pandemic – we must keep moving forward.

Chapter Fourteen

HELP!

Getting the Practical Support You Need

Is there anybody out there?

I FOUND THE SINGLE MOST frustrating thing about looking after Alan was that there was no 'one-stop shop' that would give me all the information I needed. I really hope that my experience will help you to work out what support will be most useful for you and access it accordingly. Whatever your circumstances, there will be help available, but I know that finding it can be a bewildering process. The details of lots of useful organisations are listed in Appendix Two.

In the autumn of 2017, when Alan is ready to leave the Brain Rehab Centre, I begin a series of meetings with different social workers. As has become the norm, we never see the same person twice. Things are made even more complicated by the fact that a whole extra array of social workers need to travel over from our home borough, which is on the other side of town.

The staff have done lengthy assessments and concluded that Alan is ready to leave but cannot live by himself. But he cannot come home until all the paperwork is completed. Question after question is asked, and alarmingly, we seem to be getting to a stage where I am being asked to sign some scary-looking documents confirming that Alan is mentally incompetent. No one gives any indication of the purpose of all of this form-filling, but eventually I realise that they are to do with the funding of his care. He seems to have turned from a patient to a problem. After days of discussion, the social worker asks if we have assets over £23,000. I look at him incredulously and tell him that, as he knows, we own our own home, so clearly yes, we do. He looks at me solemnly and says that in that case he is sorry to tell me that Alan won't be eligible for funding for a nursing home. I say as slowly and clearly as I possibly can that we never had any intention of putting Alan in a nursing home, and couldn't he have ascertained that at the beginning of this process? And also, maybe the question about the £23,000 of assets should come at the start rather than the end of the form?

Then we start another interminable bit of form-filling to see if I can claim a Carer's Allowance. Again, we get a long way through the paperwork before he asks if I earn more than £125 a week. I am still doing some freelance work for the publishing sales company Alan founded, so yes, I do, just. Again, he looks at me sadly, and tells me that this means I won't be eligible for a Carer's Allowance. What I need to do, he says, is apply for a Personal Independence Payment for Alan – this is the benefit for someone with a long-term illness or disability.

I go home, register on the Department for Work and Pensions (DWP) website, download the forms and begin filling in yet more complicated paperwork. Unsurprisingly, a lot of evidence is needed to prove that Alan has indeed got a permanent disability. It takes days, but eventually it is all done, and I post it off. Nothing happens.

After a week or so I finally get through on the phone to someone at the DWP to ask what is happening. A long wait while he stares at a computer screen. 'Hmm,' he says. 'I don't quite understand why this hasn't been processed.' Another long wait, and then he laughs. 'Oh, hang on,' he says. 'Of course it hasn't. Your husband is over 65. You can't get the Personal Independence Payment if you're over 65.' All of this 'computer says no' malarkey is made much worse by the fact that, at the time, I was feeling incredibly stressed and worried, as I am sure that most people applying for benefits are. Although they are pleasant enough, neither the social workers nor the DWP seem to start from the premise of actually trying to help. I conclude that once Alan comes home, we are on our own.

Attendance Allowance

However, during the process of booking Alan into a Day Respite Centre, I meet a wonderful lady there called Liz. She is friendly and chatty, and she immediately 'gets' the issues of looking after someone with a disability in a way that the bureaucrats haven't. As soon as she hears that Alan can't be left alone, she says, 'I'm sure you will qualify for the Attendance Allowance,' and offers to help me fill in the form. I am getting rather good at form-filling by this point, so I manage it by myself, but it is incredibly kind, and I feel like hugging her. She tells me that she sees relatives all the time who are so bewildered and saddened by their sudden change in circumstances that the medical jargon and legalese of the paperwork is quite beyond them.

And this time, hurrah, the DWP writes back to say that because Alan needs to be 'constantly supervised with or without short breaks through the day and night', he will qualify for a weekly payment of £85. It is an enormous relief, and apart from anything, will help pay for the one day a week when for five hours he goes to the Day Respite Centre to give me a break from looking after him.

Respite care

If you are caring for someone else with a disability, it is exhausting, and you do need a break. According to Carers UK, there are 6.5 million people in Britain who are carers; that's one in eight adults who care, unpaid, for family and friends. A survey by NHS Digital in 2017 revealed that 63.5% of carers say they have had no or not enough support. Like many people, because I felt so strongly that Alan needed to live with me, initially, the idea of him spending any time at all in any sort of 'care home' felt abhorrent. And people suffering from some sort of brain illness or injury often do seem to have an almost inbuilt fear of such places, believing them to be a slippery slope to permanent incarceration and isolation from their families. Knowing how expensive full-time residential care is, I also perceived respite care to be costly.

However, many of my assumptions were wrong. Day centres can be run by local authorities or by charities, and there are a large variety, which provide varying levels of care. Some might provide personal care and health checks or cater for people with specific issues or disabilities; others might be for older people or provide specialist care.

I find out about a place called Homelink, which is run by a

charity. When I click on their website, although it is well designed and welcoming, I nearly abandon the whole idea straight away. The people featured on it look old and odd. I can't put Alan here, I think. Not for the first time, I think *why* did this happen? How *can* my husband have gone from being an MD in a suit sitting in a flashy swivel chair and running a business, to an elderly gentleman sitting in a shabby armchair, snoozing and drooling?

Then I think, 'I must move forward.' I pick up the phone. And, as with so many situations, it is the people who make the difference. As soon as I speak to Liz, my perspective changes. She is cheerful and practical. I discover that, although some of the people at Homelink are older than Alan, plenty are younger, and they are there for all sorts of different reasons. 'Oh yes,' she says matter of factly. 'Some of our clients don't want to be here. They make no end of fuss when their carers leave them. But they have a really nice day, even though they sometimes say they haven't when it's time to go home.' We visit, and it is just as friendly and welcoming as Liz is. I discover that, thanks to generous charitable subsidies, one day a week for Alan would be affordable. And he doesn't hate it.

Three years on, he still never remembers that he goes there every Tuesday, still says he can't remember anything about it even when we're driving into the car park, and like many of the clients, his main concern as I leave is that I will remember to come and get him at 3pm. But when I do collect him, he always says he's had a good day. The staff are absolutely brilliant, and the other clients of course have plenty in common with Alan. When I see him chatting and laughing with them all, it reminds me of what a people person he is. He might think he doesn't need company, but he does, we all do.

And I have a little trick that I sometimes use when we arrive and he says, 'Oh god, look at all these nutters, do I really have to go here?' After reminding him that he is, in fact, equally nuts, I suggest that he sees it as doing his bit to help other people. By chatting to the other clients and contributing to the general cheerfulness of the place, he will be giving something back to the healthcare community that has done so much for him. At this, he usually perks up considerably; everyone likes to feel they are needed more than they are in need. Homelink is one of the best things in our life these days, and I couldn't imagine looking after Alan without their help.

'Whose patient are you again?'

When Alan finally comes home, in theory he passes smoothly from the gentle embrace of the hospital back into the arms of his own GP. In practice this is not quite how it works. First of all, there is an almost amusing battle to actually get him back onto their books. The surgery receptionist tells me initially that I can't register him, he'll have to do it himself. When I explain that this won't be possible as he has a brain injury and doesn't know where he's living, let alone who his doctor is, she sniffs. She looks at her computer and tells me she can see he's moved house to... she peers at the screen and reads out the address of the Brain Rehab Centre. Am I saying that he's now moved house again? Do I have any proof of his new address? I patiently explain that, no, he hasn't 'moved house', he was in hospital for a long, long time, and now he's come home. At no point in all this is there the slightest indication from her that the last year might have been an unusual one. In fact, the implication is that he is very lucky to be able to be accepted as a patient at this surgery at all.

Once he is signed back on with his doctor, things continue to be slightly surreal. Every couple of months, I take Alan back to hospital for a meeting with his neurology consultant, and following that meeting, she writes to Alan's doctor and sends me a copy of the letter. But whenever we see Alan's doctor to discuss flu jabs, statins, etc., she makes no reference to these letters. It is almost as if we are talking about an entirely different patient. I'm not expecting her to become an expert on encephalitis, and I know GPs are jolly busy, but there appears to be no discernible connection between the hospital and the surgery. The same confusion arises as to whether the neurologist or the GP is actually prescribing Alan's 15 pills a day. Sometimes our fabulous local pharmacist tells me that no one has prescribed them, or half the medication is available on a repeat prescription but the other half isn't. On other occasions, I arrive at the pharmacy to find an absolute glut of pills waiting behind the counter.

Keep taking the tablets

If you talk to someone about which pills they are taking, especially someone elderly, they will almost certainly say 'I've no idea what they all do' or 'I really don't know if they're doing me any good', and these remarks reveal a serious issue with 'polypharmacy' as it's called – taking lots of different pills. In 2019, Age UK conducted a study which revealed that:

...in England, more than one in ten people aged over 65 take at least eight different prescribed medications each week. It is estimated that up to 50% of all medicines for long term conditions are not taken as intended and around one in five prescriptions for older people living at home may be inappro-priate. Failing to properly manage older people's medicines is having a significant impact on their care and is making poor use of NHS resources.

To begin with, I found the number of pills that Al needed to take was highly daunting. They range from those that are frighteningly essential, such as anti-epileptic drugs to prevent his damaged brain having further seizures and steroids to dampen down his immune system to prevent the encephalitis returning, to those that are there only to counteract the effects of the other pills. I found it helpful to type up a list of everything he was taking, with a short description of the actual pill (e.g., purple lozenge) and a one-sentence summary of its purpose (e.g., antidepressant, improves motivation). It is a good idea to write the type of pill (e.g., paracetamol) as well as the brand name (e.g., Anadin). You can find all this information on the folded paper inside the pill packet. Then I arranged the list to show which pills needed to be taken and when. Apart from being an extremely useful bit of paper that you can wave at a doctor if required, I think it is also important for a patient to feel involved in their own care. Alan can't manage his own medication (and frequently doesn't even remember that he's taking any), but at least if he asks, I can explain what the function of each pill is, which I hope makes him feel more in control and less as if he is just blindly knocking back drugs when I tell him to.

Having a written summary can also prevent mistakes occur-ring. While at the Brain Rehab Centre, Alan was taken off a strong anticoagulation drug (apixaban), which he was on because he developed a blood clot that has now gone. However, the staff were not aware that he had a stent put in six years earlier and therefore should still be on some sort of blood-thinning medication. As soon as I see an actual list of medicines rather than just a little pot of pills, I notice this and get him swiftly put back onto a low dose of aspirin. This list of medications is a good thing to keep with you in a wallet or a purse, as you never know when you might need it. Take a photo of it too and keep it on your phone. There are many occasions when you may be asked about medication, when you go to the dentist for example, or if you get delayed on holiday and need to get emergency supplies, or if you have an accident and end up in A&E.

The other thing I would wholeheartedly recommend is to get a pill box with compartments for each day. They are less than £5 online or from a chemist. This means you can sort out all the different pills once a week rather than fiddling about with them every day. You can easily see if you've remembered to take the day's pills or not, and it means you can just have one small box that you can keep by your bed or in the kitchen rather than lots of packets and bottles rattling around in your handbag or cluttering up your bedroom. Trust me, it will save time, and anything that makes your house feel less like a hospital and more like a home is a good thing.

Money, money, money

Part of the process of going through any long-term illness is almost certainly going to be adjusting to finding yourself in an entirely new financial situation. Maybe you are still too ill to work. Maybe you can no longer earn an income because you are now a full-time carer for a parent or child. Maybe your ongoing health issues now involve a lot of expensive travel back and forth to a hospital. Maybe you have had to make adjustments to your home or buy special equipment. The stark fact is that any serious ailment is going to leave you considerably less well off. This may seem obvious, but it is quite a shock when it happens to you.

Once this reality sinks in, your first thought is likely to be how colossally unfair it is that you should have to cope with both sickness and financial problems at the same time. Your second thought might be: why is there no one person or organisation who can tell me everything I need to know? And your third thought might be that if I, a reasonably competent person with English as a first language, am struggling to access the labyrinthine intricacies of the UK benefits system, what on earth is it like for those who are less able than me?

A sick note

At the beginning, Alan's illness is so sudden and serious that it takes quite a while for his colleagues and many friends in the book industry to properly appreciate what is happening. This results in an amusingly wide variety of cards, many of which are hopelessly inappropriate. We're sitting in the waiting room of the ICU, opening cards that say 'Hey old buddy, I hear you're under the weather.' One features an enormous ape with the message 'Gary the Get-Well Gorilla says Cheer Up!' which at least makes us laugh, a lot.

Even now, years later, it is clear that his clients and colleagues truly miss him. He was always a people person, a hands-on boss, happy to chat at any time, much more of a man for phone calls or meetings in person rather than emails, and his team of reps all spoke to him most days. Publishers also called him up whenever they needed to; many is the time the kids heard their dad sorting out an issue with supply to WHSmith or Waterstones while we were driving down a French autoroute or sitting in a Cornish car park. From the moment he went into hospital, for colleagues and clients alike, there was complete silence.

For the reps whose jobs are solitary, and the small independent publishers who are used to frequent friendly reassurance, I can tell this leaves a horrible gap. I realise that although I've lost a husband, losing a boss, a mentor and a colleague is also extremely difficult.

In July, Alan's sick pay comes to an abrupt end. Alan has been the main breadwinner in our home for many years, and the financial adjustment to our lives on top of coping with his illness was just not something I was prepared for. A relatively quick conversation with the DWP confirms that a fairly affluent, home-owning, some-savings-in-the-bank employee of 67 who is off ill for longer than 28 weeks is not entitled to anymore sick pay. Which is fair enough but was a big shock, nonetheless. We were incredibly lucky in that we had some savings to live on, partly because Alan's father had died the year before. And we had nearly paid off our mortgage. But the combination of increased costs plus vastly reduced income is a sucker punch that hits many families when the main earner falls ill.

The benefits of benefits

One important thing to take on board early on is that being in receipt of one benefit tends to act as a 'certifier' for another. So, my advice would be that if you are eligible for anything, you must claim it. Even if you feel you don't need it. This is because if you don't claim one benefit, you will find it a great deal harder to claim other benefits, as 'the system' will assume you aren't eligible. A prime example is getting a discount on your council tax. Although the rules only state that you must be *eligible* for benefits, many councils (including mine) will ask for proof that you are *receiving* the benefit. A similar thing happens with student loans – see below.

Power of attorney (POA)

This is undoubtably the bit of paper that enables you to help another person the most. For nearly two years I resisted even starting the process of applying for the POA, which would empower me to make legal decisions on Alan's behalf. The doctors were happy for me to make welfare decisions as Alan's wife, and since all our finances are held jointly, I didn't need any extra authority to manage things at home. To me, it symbolised something frighteningly finite, and I wasn't ready to acknowledge that never again would Alan be able to manage his own life.

A POA is a formidable document, but what I didn't originally appreciate is that there are different types, you can set up different requirements for health and financial decisions, more than one 'agent' can hold it for the same person, it can be revoked and you don't have to use it once you have it – i.e., where at all possible, I can still let Alan make his own decisions. The truly sensible thing to do is set it up (as many solicitors advise) when you are in perfect health, and you can decide at leisure who you would like to manage your affairs if you are not able to. If you are a carer for someone, you will undoubtably need a POA at some point (for me, the moment arrived when I tried to sort out

Alan's pension) and you will need a solicitor to help you, as the wording and the rules are complex. But it does make many of the practicalities of caring much easier. Like the magic ID card that Doctor Who uses to flash at the authorities on alien planets, it will open many doors and ensure you are taken seriously.

Council tax reduction

I am sitting in my kitchen, having lunch with Al a few months after he's come out of hospital, when suddenly a text pings in from Lucy. She's listening to Radio 4, and they are talking about the fact that if you have someone living with you who is 'severely mentally impaired', you are eligible for a 25% reduction in your council tax. The point of the Radio 4 feature is to raise awareness that councils tend not to advertise this fact, because they don't really want people to claim it. Sure enough, despite the fact that I am now quite 'embedded' in the benefits system, absolutely no one has mentioned this to me.

I check it out online and discover that this is correct. A major investigation by MoneySavingExpert.com in 2017 revealed that tens of thousands of vulnerable people are likely to be missing out 'in all likelihood due to inappropriate information being given about the discount by local councils'. Two-thirds of those councils they surveyed 'gave incorrect info, while some frontline staff were apparently unaware of the existence of the discount'. If the person you live with has 'a severe impairment of intelligence and social functioning (however caused) which appears to be permanent' then you qualify. It doesn't matter whether it's caused by encephalitis, Parkinson's, dementia, Alzheimer's, a tumour or an accident. And it doesn't matter how much your house is worth or if you have any savings, although some councils may try to tell you that it does. In fact, if you are living alone with a severe mental impairment (SMI), then you qualify for a 100% reduction i.e., you shouldn't be paying *any* council tax!

In order to receive the reduction, Alan has to be eligible for one of a number of benefits, which he is, and I need his neurology consultant to certify that he has a SMI, which she is happy to do. The council drag their feet on sending me the relevant forms and then make a bit of a hash of applying the reduction to my standing order, but thanks to Lucy, we get the benefit of this significant saving – around £400 a year.

Student finance

A charity puts me in touch with a lovely lady whose husband has also had encephalitis. She tells me she is 'quite the terrier' when it comes to making sure she gets the benefits that are due to her, and she is the first person to mention to me that due to our change in circumstances, we may well be eligible for some extra help with funding Madeleine's university education; she was halfway through her first year when Alan fell ill.

I check it out, and although the rules have changed over the years since 1998 when students first started paying for their own education (and they may well change again), essentially, she is correct, and I am very grateful to her for thinking of it. The situation in England is currently that if a family's income is below £25,000 per annum, they can get a much larger student loan. In essence, the student can borrow all the money they should need for accommodation and living costs, which is roughly £9000 pa (in addition to the loan for the tuition fees). (If your family income is above £60,000, they can borrow about half of this, which is where we were before Alan got ill.)

Crucially, this is a loan not a grant, and with repayment interest rates at 6%, you might question whether saddling the poorest students with the largest debt is really a very good idea. However, only by claiming the maximum loan will students be eligible for any additional financial help that the universities themselves may offer. This was the case with Madeleine. The bursary from Warwick was very helpful and, unlike the loan, didn't need to be repaid.

Charitable help

While Alan is still in hospital, I get a chatty text on his phone from a publicist friend of his who doesn't know he's been ill. She does a lot of work for The Book Trade Charity, a well-known organisation within the publishing industry who have many fundraising events and parties that Alan has often attended. She is aghast when she hears about Alan's situation and offers lots of sympathy. Then, a day later, she sends a follow-up text, suggesting that if we need any financial assistance, the charity may well be able to help. I stare at it, horrified. Charity! We don't need charity thanks very much, I think. I'm still convinced at this point that Alan will make a full recovery and return to work.

Fast forward a year, and I remember her kind suggestion and get back in touch. And they couldn't be kinder or more helpful. By far the hardest bit was putting aside my embarrassment at asking for help in the first place. Everyone knows what a marvellous thing our NHS is, but I believe that the network of charities that we have in the UK is just as amazing, and how much they contribute to the nation's health is much less acknowledged. Certainly, at the point when Alan was leaving the care of the Brain Rehab Centre, I was completely unaware of how important their role was to become to us.

When you leave hospital, you can feel very vulnerable, especially if, like Alan, you have been inside for a long time. Officially, you are returning to the care of your GP, but in reality, that is not what we found. Instead, we were scooped up and carried onwards by a whole range of charitable organisations, and without them, we would have struggled. If you want to boost our healthcare system, I think one of the most useful things you can do is support one of the thousands of charities that bolster it up. Below are my three superheroes (further details are listed in Appendix Two) but, of course, the big ones such as Macmillan Cancer Support or Children in Need may be your personal saviours. And the smaller ones that are local to you may be the most helpful of all – there is a wonderful community gym near us, for example, which runs supervised sessions and has been invaluable for helping Alan's physical recovery.

Encephalitis Society

This is a brilliant charity, who have helped us enormously. As *The Guardian* journalist Simon Hattenstone writes, the CEO of the Encephalitis Society, Dr Ava Easton, has 'taken what was a deadly but obscure illness out to the world and explained it simply and cogently to people who have no reason to have thought about it before and to experts who almost certainly never thought about it in those terms before'.

Headway: The Brain Injury Association

It was the NHS therapists in the hospital who pointed us towards Headway, and we met with Fiona in the hospital coffee shop, long before Alan was ready to come home. Through its network of groups and branches across the UK, it provides support, services and information. I went to my first Headway meeting by myself, and sitting in a church hall and telling our story to a circle of sympathetic listeners was massively therapeutic.

Illness and injury are shockingly random, and this charity helps a wide range of people of all ages and with all sorts of brain trauma. I met people who had been left with brain damage because of infection or disease certainly, but also from a car accident or a violent attack. I think it showed me that it is good to keep an open mind about where you may find common ground, and I found it beneficial to meet other people whose lives had been turned upside down like ours by the dramatic speed of a brain injury. The good thing about Headway is that they are a big network and can put you in touch with others. Joining a group or meeting up on a one-to-one basis with other people in the same position as you doesn't suit everyone, but I think it's a good thing to try, to see if it helps.

Integrated Neurological Services (INS)

INS is a charity, founded 25 years ago by an experienced physiotherapist who identified the gap in long-term support and education for people with neurological conditions and their carers and which aims 'to develop their self-reliance, enable them to live as independently as possible and thus enhance their quality of life'. It can be a bit of a trek for me to get Alan there, but it is always worth it. One of the biggest issues facing us when Alan came out of rehab was: what was he actually going to do with himself all day? Because he needs someone with him all the time and can't travel by himself, most 'hobby-type' activities were not appropriate. At INS he has done gardening classes, Tai Chi, exercise, counselling, music, physio and more. Some of the most successful activities have been the simplest, for example the 'Vintage TV Comedy' session. Watching old clips of sitcoms and comedians and laughing your head off for an afternoon in the company of others – what's not to like? I had no idea such charities existed before Alan got ill, but now I know that these organisations are a lifeline for many. The best thing about them is that their relatively small size means that they offer personal, friendly and practical solutions without being weighed down by bureaucracy, but at the same time, they are run by a team of very well-qualified professionals. I'm sure there are many organisations like INS all around the country, and they really do need more recognition for the vital services they provide.

INS tell me that patients with neurological conditions have the lowest health-related quality of life of any long-term condition, and much of what they do is aimed at reducing loneliness and depression, which contributes to improved wellbeing in patients and carers. They have certainly made an enormous difference to Alan and me.

Chapter Fifteen

THE BIG QUESTIONS

I need answers

ONE OF THE THINGS I found hardest about the way that illness derailed our ordinary life was that it threw up so many questions. Aside from the purely practical – Will Alan get better? What will we do for money? How do I tell people? – and the emotional issues around fear and grief, there were also the more philosophical doubts: what's the point of it all? Is there an afterlife? Do we matter? Milan Kundera, in his wonderful novel *The Unbearable Lightness of Being*, wrote:

> Indeed, the only truly serious questions are ones that even a child can formulate. Only the most naive of questions are truly serious. They are the questions with no answers. A question with no answer is a barrier that cannot be breached. In other words, it is questions with no answers that set the limit of human possibilities, describe the boundaries of human existence.

I think this perfectly describes what happens when someone

falls seriously ill. As well as addressing the small and personal problems of humanity, it also makes you think deeply about larger existential uncertainties.

What if?

Perhaps the biggest question we ask ourselves when someone falls ill is: What could have happened? What if I'd gone to the doctor sooner? What if my child hadn't been running for that bus? What if my mum hadn't ignored that lump? What if my dad hadn't been a smoker? And then: What if the consultants are wrong? What if the doctor has made a mistake? What if another hospital is better? What if I get a second opinion? What if I'd been treated faster? For us, initially there were the questions as to whether we'd missed some vital warning sign about Alan's health. We collectively racked our brains and were all 100% sure we hadn't, which made us feel better. However, I'm pretty sure that even if there had been signs, for example if Alan had been more tired and forgetful in the run-up to his first seizure or even if there had been some downright odd behaviour, we probably wouldn't have done anything differently. We're not a family of hypochondriacs, and in general, I believe that has served us well.

When someone is ill, people kindly say, 'You did everything you could,' but that's almost certainly not true; there are always things you could have done differently, done better. Rather than either pushing that thought to the back of your mind, or worse still, torturing yourself with it, I think you can learn to accept that a big 'what if' can just stay dangling there. People quite often ask me whether the permanent brain injury that Alan now has could have been avoided. And logically, the answer must be yes.

If, after the first seizure, the medics had rushed him into hospital, put him onto the plasma exchange machine and removed the 'bad' antibodies (which were causing his brain to malfunction) from his blood, or given him a large shot of Rituximab (which also zaps the GABA B antibodies), I guess he might have made a full recovery. But that would have required a speed and accuracy of diagnosis of literally superhuman proportions. And medically, the consequences of that course of action if it *hadn't* been autoimmune encephalitis (99% more likely) would have been catastrophic.

Letting those 'what if' questions run riot in your head is not helpful, but I know it's all too easy to do. I read about many cases in hospitals where a family is endlessly trying to rewind what has happened and then fast forward to a better outcome. What I found more productive was to turn the big 'what if' round the other way and hypothesise how very easily things could have been considerably worse. What if Alan had had his seizure 48 hours earlier when he was driving us down the motorway? What if he'd got encephalitis ten years earlier, before some clever scientist came up with the test for the GABA B antibodies? What if we didn't live in a country with access to one of the best healthcare services in the world? What if he didn't have a family like ours to look after him?

I should be so lucky?

Believing you are lucky rather than unlucky can certainly influence how you feel about being ill, but can it have an actual effect on your health? An article in *The Guardian* quotes a study (2016) saying that 'believing in chance may just make you luckier'. Dr

Mike Aitken, from Cambridge University, says that 'research has suggested that people who think of themselves as lucky actually are lucky'. A 'belief in good luck scale' study developed in 1997 by two Canadian psychologists showed that 'those who believe they are inherently lucky tend to be of an optimistic bent, and a seemingly lucky event – a "lucky break" – made them even more confident and optimistic.' Is this helpful in hospital?

Historically, medicine has always been closely associated with superstition. The Greek physician Hippocrates (in around 400 BC) is generally credited with being the person responsible for separating medicine from religion and believing that diseases were caused by environmental factors, diet and living habits and were not a punishment inflicted by the gods. However, for the next two millennia, many societies and cultures still attributed many of the causes and cures of disease to magic and the divine. While modern scientific medicine rejects any supernatural origin for disease, lots of patients still hold superstitious beliefs or have dangerous misconceptions about where certain diseases come from. For example, the idea that witchcraft can cause and heal diseases is still widespread within developing countries, especially in Africa. Research has shown that an irrational belief in things that bring 'bad luck' tends to have a very poor effect on a society's health. One study (2019) looking at a belief in ghosts in Taiwan found that 'this type of false belief has far-reaching consequences not only for health-related behaviour, but also for health outcomes and even for mortality'.

But what about a link between a belief in *good* luck and health outcomes? An interesting article in *The New York Times* (2006) asked, 'In science-based medicine, where does luck fit in?' It wonders 'why doctors and patients are so reluctant to discuss a phenomenon that permeates medicine every day'. A doctor hypothesises that 'a more frank acknowledgment of the role luck plays' might be helpful. He points out that 'some patients who are 100% compliant with their doctors' wishes will still die' and that clearly 'these are the unlucky ones. And then there are always those patients who constantly disregard medical recommendations and seemingly suffer no ill effects. You guessed it: lucky.'

But can a patient influence their own luck? Studies have shown that people perform better on tasks when they have a lucky charm with them, so might this also be the case if the 'task' in question is recovery? Psychologist Stuart Vyse says that 'lucky charms create an illusion of control for the person who believes in them'. 'Even though many people might not know how their lucky charms actually work, it is not a bad idea to carry a charm for added confidence, it is a "low cost" belief,' says Professor Maia Young. In other words, it won't do any harm and might well do some good. An article in *Medical News Today* tells me that a belief in superstitions 'can have a soothing effect, relieving anxiety about the unknown and giving people a sense of control over their lives'. *The International Journal of Psychology and Behavioral Sciences* found that although superstitions produce 'a false sense of having control over outer conditions', they genuinely 'can reduce anxiety'.

It certainly seems to be the case that seeing yourself as lucky rather than cursed will make a difference to the way you move through life. Psychologist Courtney E. Ackerman says that the many benefits of cultivating a positive mindset 'include better overall health, better ability to cope with stress, and greater well-being.' As Alan recovered, frequently telling him that he was lucky – to have a family that could look after him, not to be in a wheelchair, to be alive – definitely had a positive effect on his mood, and mine too.

As a family, we are not especially superstitious, but when

I thought about it, I realised we are much more likely to refer to good luck rather than bad luck. So, walking under ladders, magpies, putting umbrellas up indoors or the number 13 hold no sway over us, but we have quite a few little oddities that we think of as good omens. One is if we hear a Paul Simon song on the radio. This started years ago when I was taking one of the children to a music exam, and we heard *You Can Call Me Al* in the car, just before we arrived. They did well in the exam, and then on the way to the next violin exam about a year later, the same thing happened and again they did well. Over the years, we've heard Paul Simon songs before GCSEs, football matches, driving tests and all manner of other stressful occasions and always we think 'that's the good luck' – sometimes texting each other to pass it on. I'm sure lots of families have such traditions, and although I don't believe there is some omnipotent power up above deciding when to play *50 Ways to Leave Your Lover* to us, I do think that the small boost that hearing the song provides can sometimes be enough to positively influence the situation.

Believing yourself to be lucky can certainly affect your mental health, and there's no question that your mental health has an effect on your physical health. It was astonishingly bad luck that Alan got autoimmune encephalitis. Nothing seems to have caused it – just a glitch in his immune system. But it was very lucky that he was surrounded by people who could look after him, and acknowledging this has certainly helped his recovery.

Does 'what doesn't kill you make you stronger'?

This was Nietzsche's opinion, and it is frequently quoted as a mantra for helping you get through tough times. Ernest

Hemingway wrote that 'we are stronger in the places we've been broken', which has a similarly macho tone, implying that pain and trauma are good for us. But is this true? Some Christian thinking centres on the idea that 'trial and tribulation' will make you a better person. People can feel that being challenged by hardship is a test – either from God or just from life in general. The apostle Paul wrote that 'suffering produces endurance, and endurance produces character; and character produces hope' (*Romans 5:3,4*), but clearly that isn't always true. I am not entirely convinced about the idea of adversity as a trial that must be overcome and will make you into a better person. A commonly used metaphor for this concept is the example of a tree, which when buffeted by storms, puts down deeper and deeper roots. Eventually, the tree that has withstood many tempests will be a tougher tree than the one that has grown in more clement climes. What hasn't killed it has, in fact, made it stronger.

Every week, while Alan is doing physio at a special gym, I walk in a huge park, and halfway round my regular route is a large oak tree that has been blown over and now lies completely on its side. At first sight, you cannot work out how it has continued to grow. All its branches are on one side, but they shoot upwards with bushy vigour and strength, each now looking like its own small tree sprouting from the sturdy trunk, which has been worn smooth from people sitting, playing and climbing on it. When you look closely, you see that although almost all its roots are exposed, some of them have managed to cling on to the earth and supply the oak with enough energy to flourish. This tree has not grown stronger, but it has grown differently; it has adapted and become something new. This is the tree for me, and every time I see it, it makes me feel heartened.

Do the drugs work?

Near the beginning, a calm, softly spoken doctor sits next to my sleeping husband and takes me through the options for treating the different types of encephalitis. She explains that if it is caused by an infection then it will be relatively straightforward, but if it is autoimmune encephalitis then it will be 'not easy – much more difficult'. She explains that they will need to do many more tests and try many different combinations of medication before they know what will work. I don't want to hear 'much more difficult'. I want Alan to have an MRI scan so the doctors can find something wrong in his brain and then get rid of it. I think it's often the same with a diagnosis of cancer – the solution in our heads is 'cut that bastard out, annihilate those evil cells'. It's an almost primal response that does modern medicine a huge disservice. The doctor explains that despite major progress, brain surgery is still pretty basic and rarely the solution. The real advances over the last decades have been in treating brains with drugs, not scalpels.

I've come to realise over the years since that conversation that an ignorance (and often downright scepticism) about the effectiveness of modern medication is shared by many. An 'I'm not sure if pills really do any good' mentality is prevalent, coupled with a fear of 'Big Pharma' and the nagging thought that doctors are in the pockets of the drug companies, trying to get as many of us hooked on unnecessary tablets as they can. This has surely contributed to the truly alarming fear of vaccines. As reported in *The Guardian* (2019), figures from the World Health Organization show that measles cases worldwide rose by 300% during the first three months of 2019 compared with 2018, largely attributed to the impact of anti-vaccination campaigns. Another worrying trend is the rise in those turning their back on 'the science stuff' in treating cancer. I see in *The Telegraph* (2019) a tragic story of a patient whose:

> ...2a triple negative breast cancer was diagnosed...and was offered a mastectomy, chemotherapy and radiotherapy. But she rejected conventional therapy in favour of a vegan diet of mainly raw fruit and vegetables, supplemented with turmeric, seaweed and spells in a hyperbaric oxygen chamber.

She died. Many of the things that I, family, friends and therapists have done over the years since Alan had encephalitis have undoubtably helped him, but it is science that has kept him alive.

Shall I tell you a story?

When I worked in a primary school, we used to teach pupils how to write stories with a clear beginning, middle and end. One of the hardest things is realising that illness is not at all like how it is portrayed in films or books. There is no arc, no climax, no resolution, and you never know which chapter of the story you have reached. Lots of people have said to me that they are pleased I am writing a book about my experiences because 'something good will come out of something bad', but I understand why that can also be a misleading and maybe hurtful statement, and I acknowledge my children's worries that I might 'neaten' what has happened into a narrative with a start and finish that it doesn't have.

Dr Sarosh Irani, an expert in autoimmune encephalitis, believes that 'more attention to patient narratives will assist in future clinical research studies to further improve outcomes'. The neurologist Oliver Sacks, in the introduction to his wise and funny book on brain disorders, *The Man Who Mistook His Wife for a Hat*, says that he is hoping to revive the 'tradition of richly human clinical tales...in the hope that others might learn and understand'. Of course, I am no neurologist, but my hope is the same. I loved Rachel Clarke's book *Dear Life: A Doctor's Story of Love and Loss*, and especially the paragraph where she says that:

> Storytelling is the bedrock of good medical practice... It is undeniable that the meanings we construct around our affliction and diseases, the stories we tell ourselves about what is wrong and where we are heading, can overturn our experience of illness.[1]

That's what I feel too, but I know the children are concerned that my book will become the only narrative, the 'true story'. If anything, I hope that this book will help people see that there are many alternative stories to be told about one illness.

When I was 16, my beloved Grannie Pinkerton died, after a summer of cancer, and it was easily the saddest thing that had ever happened to me. I was on holiday with my younger siblings and cousins at the time, and I mostly kept my misery to myself. So much so that I remember my littlest cousin Keith, who was eight, saying to me that he and the other younger members of the family couldn't understand why I wasn't weeping like them, and maybe I didn't care, which of course I found very hurtful. But at the same time, I gave no thought at all to the feelings of my mum and auntie who had been in and out of hospital day after day to sit by the bedside of their dying mother. Those three experiences

---

1   Reproduced from *Dear Life: A Doctor's Story of Love and Loss* by Rachel Clarke with permission from Little, Brown Book Group (UK) and Aitken Alexander on behalf of Thomas Dunne Books (US).

of Grannie P's death are equally 'true', but I expect if I ask my dad or siblings what their memories of that time are, I will get other, different stories. As Julian Barnes says in *The Sense of an Ending*, his Booker prize-winning meditation on recollection and regret, 'What you end up remembering isn't always the same as what you have witnessed.' Talking about our experiences can hopefully help us all to make sense of what happened, and I certainly see my story as just one patch in a whole quilt of memories and truths.

In her remarkable book *Life After Encephalitis*, which gives a voice to the stories of many encephalitis survivors, Dr Ava Easton writes that 'Narratives are an integral and important element in modern society. Their use in medicine reflects a changing relationship between patient and doctor.' She goes on to suggest that the 'lost tradition of narrative' is being revived in the teaching and practice of medicine around the world and that 'supporters believe that patients' narratives will provide education which enriches the health professional's understanding and expands their treatment toolkit'.

Has 'He' got the whole world in his hands?

Finding yourself in a hospital situation is when many people frequently also 'find God'. People will tell you they have never prayed so hard for anything as when their child was struggling for life, and lots of us know that feeling of offering up a quiet 'thank you' to the heavens when an operation has gone well or a worst-case scenario hasn't happened. Many of us make silent bargains with God, promising never to ask for anything ever again if He will just make things alright – I know I did.

The problem with hoping that your prayers will be answered

is that, rationally, you have to wonder what that means if they aren't. Which puts things into stark relief – at the start of Alan's illness we were praying for a complete recovery, not permanent brain damage. It is very easy to see how people lose their faith. As Stephen Fry famously put it, 'Why should I respect a capricious, mean-minded, stupid God who creates a world that is so full of injustice and pain?' There's plenty in the Bible telling us that God is listening to us, but what happens if there's no response – does that mean that children die because their parents didn't go to church or pray hard enough? The Bible also talks a lot about God's will, but the idea that it is somehow God's decision that someone you love should suffer is pretty unbearable. After the terrorist bombing of the Manchester Arena, I heard a man saying on the radio (2017) that his niece had escaped uninjured because 'she had a guardian angel looking down on her', and I found myself crying with fury at the suggestion that the other children who died had therefore been abandoned by the angels. It is very hard to reconcile the idea of God as protector of the innocent with an acknowledgement that innocents will die nonetheless.

But an older friend said to me that when her husband had been ill, she had found a lot of comfort in her belief that he was 'in God's hands', and oddly enough, I found that idea extremely helpful. I think it is because it took away the pressure to feel that I had to try and control the situation. Once I accepted that I couldn't necessarily alter the future, it made me feel a lot calmer. Realising that there are limits to what we humans can achieve can give you permission to pray and hope but without the agony of feeling that you have personally failed if things don't work out. I don't know if prayers work but neither do Richard Dawkins, Alan's doctor or the Archbishop of Canterbury. The fact that we don't know what tomorrow will bring is paradoxically the one fact that atheists and those who are religious can all agree on. No one can truly predict the outcome of illness, and accepting that uncertainty can bring peace.

You also don't need to believe in it to get something from religion that is beneficial. Many people find that going into a church or listening to hymns and prayers is both uplifting and soothing. Most hospitals have a chapel or a multi-faith room for reflection or prayer, which can be a very calming place to be. One Sunday, early on, I went to church and one of the hymns happened to be *He Who Would Valiant Be*, also known as *To Be a Pilgrim*. John Bunyan wrote the words during his 12-year prison sentence for refusing to conform to the official state church, and I found a lot of consolation in its steadfast message about battling adversity, 'No foes shall stay his might; though he with giants fight.' Many people have found the words of Psalm 23, 'even though I walk through the valley of the shadow of death, I will fear no evil, for you are with me; your rod and your staff, they comfort me', extremely consoling.

Are doctors a higher species?

I read an article in *The Guardian* that quotes TV drama writer Jed Mercurio, a former doctor himself, who says that medical dramas ignore the cynicism that infiltrates their work. I think this is true. Anyone who ever meets a medic out of a hospital environment can be struck by how black their humour is, how brutal their conversation and how jaded their world view. With a few exceptions, the doctors you see on TV screens don't remotely tally with people you meet at parties or have as friends. But of course, when you encounter a medical professional in hospital,

you see someone different again. Or rather, you don't see someone, because you don't really want to. As doctor turned author
and comedian Adam Kay says:

> Patients don't actually think of doctors as being human. It's
> why they're so quick to complain if we make a mistake or
> if we get cross. It's why they'll bite our heads off when we
> finally call them into our over-running clinic room at 7 pm,
> not thinking that we also have homes we'd rather be at. But
> it's the flip side of not wanting your doctor to be fallible,
> capable of getting your diagnosis wrong.[2]

I think he's dead right about this. As patients, we're actually
hoping that our doctor is a benevolent and omnipotent god who
can solve everything. When we say to our doctors 'What's the
prognosis?', what we're really saying is, 'Universe, what is The
Plan?' This is clearly unreasonable. Although they are extremely
well qualified, doctors can't know everything. As Adam Kay
also says, 'Human beings make mistakes and get sick and get
sad and get angry.' Having a doctor, like having a parent, is a lot
better than not having one, and they are doing their best. Good
enough is OK. Flawed, tired parents who sometimes screw up
are perfectly fine. As are doctors.

Does life matter?

During one long Sunday afternoon in hospital, sitting next to

---

2   Reproduced from *This is Going to Hurt* by Adam Kay (copyright © Adam Kay 2017)
     with permission from Pan Macmillan through PLSclear.

Alan who is asleep, I watch a patient die, right in front of me. The middle-aged man in the bed opposite is sitting up in bed, hooked up to a breathing tube, his eyes closed. Suddenly, silently, his eyes open and he paws ineffectually at his oxygen mask. Just as I am wondering what to do, a nurse notices him and calls his name urgently several times before pressing a button on the wall. Within moments, the ward is full of people, and just as in a TV drama, CPR is attempted, a defibrillator is used, time checks are given – one minute, two minutes, ten minutes. The blue curtains are swiftly swished around him, but the forceful sounds of attempted resuscitation and urgent instruction continue. Then silence. I hear the doctor asking for the family to be called, and about ten minutes later, a great many relatives arrive. Weeping, wailing, sobbing. It is deeply shocking, and I am crying too. I can't really process what has happened; it's all been so fast. The chasm between what was an ordinary afternoon and something utterly out of the ordinary is impossible to comprehend. Is that it?

What does life mean? And how can we make our lives meaningful? Dickens once wrote that 'no one is useless in this world who lightens the burdens of another', and something Christie Watson says in her book about nursing also strikes a chord with me: 'I like the idea that I can help provide meaning to another person's life, and during the same process search for meaning in my own.'

Is 'looking after your own' important?

I'm sitting in a coffee shop with a lady who I shall call 'Sally', whose husband has also had a brain injury. She is full of outrage for the way the NHS has treated her. Some of her story is very similar to mine. Like me, she has been married to her husband for a long time. Like me, she is still coming to terms with the fact that he is now a totally different person. Like me, she can notice something is wrong with him before the doctors can. Like me, she has probably spent months of her life sitting in waiting rooms and A&E departments. But her strategy has been to battle the system with a bruising belligerence. She has fallen out with almost every doctor she has come across; scores of council officials and other political bureaucrats now seem to be involved in the many issues she has, and she is taking action against the hospital for misdiagnosis and poor care.

At first, I am concerned that she has been badly advised. I have come across the 'ambulance chasing' side of the legal profession myself and worry that she might be a pawn in a solicitor's quest for compensation. Then I realise that this is not the case, and she is not trying to get any money. Fighting, writing letters, arguing with people is what she enjoys. Her eyes light up when she speaks of it; she tells me that frankly she relishes it far more than looking after her husband, which is monotonous and draining. She sees it as her job, says that it keeps her from going completely mad.

Listening to her, it is hard to tell whether the outcomes for her husband have been better or worse than if she were easier to deal with. Who is to say whether her approach or mine is the more successful one? And more successful for whom? It certainly seems to be working for her; she tells me she doesn't need any counselling, doesn't want to see herself as a victim. I admire her total certainty, her willingness to take on any fight. But then I hear of the nurses she's been rude to, the queues she's jumped, the other patients she's suggesting are bed-blocking, the council workers she's shouted at and I'm not so certain. She's looking after her husband for sure, but how far should we take 'taking care of your own' at the expense of the rest of society?

How real are memories?

I read an article about a woman who has lost her memory due to eclampsia while giving birth. A massive seizure has starved her brain of oxygen, and like Alan, she now has virtually no short-term memory and her long-term memories are patchy. Again, like Alan, she can look at photographs of herself at an event, and even if the event is an important one, like her wedding, she has no memory of the occasion whatsoever. The article is written by her husband, and one phrase really resonates with me: 'I know more about her life than she does. It's sometimes hard to wrap my head around that.'

I know exactly what he means; it is incredibly hard to process that thought. Large chunks of Alan's life are to be forever unknown. There will be things he has done, thoughts he's had, experiences he's gone through that are lost forever. It's like the philosophical question that asks whether, if no one sees a tree fall, does it actually fall? I feel acutely responsible for making sure that Alan actually does exist, that what he does has meaning and that it's documented. He never expresses an urge to look back or forward. Left to his own devices, he would undoubtedly just sleep, rest, chat and read; he is entirely happy living in the present.

Sometimes I wish we had a Pensieve for Alan to dip into – the magical dish from the *Harry Potter* books that allows characters to examine their own memories. But of course, we don't, and when I help him write his diary at the end of the day, he has usually already forgotten what's happened. As I remind him, it's an unnerving thought that I could make up the day's events and he'd probably obediently type them in, so already the memories would be false ones. If the two of us are out together and something nice happens, it's unsettling to realise that I'll be the only one to remember it. And it's the same with all the shared memories we had from when we were first together or when the children were little. I'm the sole guardian of those memories now – there's no one to corroborate or challenge them, and that can be awfully hard to deal with.

In *The Sense of an Ending*, Julian Barnes writes that 'History is that certainty produced at the point where the imperfections of memory meet the inadequacies of documentation.' And sometimes it does feel as if I am, very inadequately, creating Alan's history.

Is life fair?

I remember, a long time ago, reading a piece by the American satirical writer P. J. O'Rourke, whose young daughter continually piped up, 'It's not fair.' He said that he'd told her in no uncertain terms that she should be jolly glad that 'it' wasn't fair, because if society operated on a more equal basis, she would be considerably less well off. It was funny, because that's a harsh thing to tell a ten-year-old, but the truth of it still strikes me whenever I or any of my friends have a bit of a middle-class moan about our first-world problems.

As Alan moved through the healthcare system, it became increasingly obvious that he was in a very good position to get excellent care; he lived near one of the best hospitals in the world, he was seriously ill but with a wife who was persistent enough to make sure he accessed everything available to him and his overall health was pretty good. If he'd been on his own, he'd have been in trouble. And a bit like Yossarian in *Catch-22*, if he'd been any crazier, he might have been too crazy to get help; the doctors needed to be certain that this was a patient who would respond well to treatment.

Of course, some might say that since Alan had worked hard and paid taxes for over 40 years, he deserved every bit of the immense amount of money that the NHS has undoubtably spent on treating him. But it is evident to anyone passing through the healthcare system in this country that, often, those who need most get least. People's health is hugely affected by where they live, their race, their occupational status and their socio-economic position, and all of these were in Alan's favour. The healthcare system in the UK is one of the best in the world, but it is not always fair. The long time we spent in hospital clarified a determination to ensure we would try to pass through the system as honestly as we possibly could.

Should illness be marketed?

I hear a woman on the radio talking about her campaign to stop the pink ribbon being used as a symbol for breast cancer charities as it 'infantilises and diminishes' it. Audrey Birt, who founded Breakthrough Breast Cancer in Scotland, says:

> Cancer isn't fun, pretty, sexy or pink but a physically exhausting and emotionally draining disease that screws your mind, takes you to the darkest places and, like a nuclear bomb, has

long-term fallout. It's lonely, isolating and bloody scary at best. At worst it's a killer.

She feels that 'the pink ribbon represents what many people would like me and other patients to be – pretending that it's all OK'. I think she has a valid point, and it clarifies my own unease at some of the images used in charity marketing campaigns for various diseases. The cute children chosen for their huge smiles, the photogenically fragile, the wanly weary, the bravely battling and the strikingly shaven; all of these patients are pictured ad nauseam, often with the insidious teeny tiny asterisk indicating *posed by models. If something more graphic is used, it's in order to shock rather than make us empathise. Sometimes it all seems a bit close to the scene in *Slumdog Millionaire* where the gang masters decide that the sweet little children begging would make even more money if they were disabled. Websites and adverts rarely show the sheer grinding boredom of illness, the unpleasantness of colostomy bags, syringes, adult nappies, bedpans and sick bowls; the patients whose ailments may have made them grumpy, irritable or overweight.

It seems reasonable to question exactly why you would want to put a positive spin on a horrible disease. Perhaps one reason might be to encourage more awareness and support. This can be especially helpful where the illness has 'shameful' or embarrassing connotations, and I think most people would agree that changing perceptions is very worthwhile if it means patients don't suffer in silence. Like Alzheimer's or dementia, encephalitis can be frightening to witness and some feel that that the 'image problem' of the illness is the reason why there isn't more help or funding.

The Encephalitis Society use a red brain for their logo, but it's not a scarily inflamed brain, it's one made up from pieces of a jigsaw, with a smiley face. Marie Curie, who offer care and support for those with terminal illnesses, use a yellow daffodil with its associations of hope, springtime and joy. The use of the pink ribbon to raise awareness of breast cancer has surely led to far more support than it would have done if they'd used, say, a black skull. The origin of the pink ribbon as a 'logo' is usually attributed to a marketing campaign by cosmetics queen Estée Lauder in 1992, launched to 'recognise an urgent need to bring breast cancer to the forefront and put a spotlight on this world health issue'. Some sources say it was also inspired by the use of a peach ribbon by American breast-cancer survivor Charlotte Haley. It has clearly been hugely successful, appearing on clothing, make-up, sportswear, soft toys, key rings and more. The Guide Dogs for the Blind Association is another example of a charity where an appealing image has caused the funds to pour in. The vision of a gorgeous golden retriever leading an angelic child off to school or guiding an elderly gentleman to the shops is an appealing one, and many other charities trying to fundraise for the visually impaired have been angered by the fact that while they struggle, this charity has millions of pounds in reserve. A spokesperson for the association itself admitted, 'People give to dogs, not to blind people.'

The opinions of patients vary greatly as to how they feel the 'image' of their illness affects them, with some like Audrey Birt saying that she feels the pink ribbon contributes to the 'pressure to cover up your scars and put on the pretty scarf, the make-up, the smile and pretend that all is well', while others believe the campaign has given them 'the confidence to talk about cancer without feeling depressed and afraid' and agree with breast cancer survivor Lindsay Nicholson, who said in *The Daily Mail* that the millions that have been raised for cancer research would never have happened without the 'recognisable and trusted' little pink ribbon, which is the colour of 'dawn, a new day, and hope'.

The truth is that illness is messy and complex, so perhaps it's unsurprising that questions about how it should be marketed are messy and complex too. PR, branding, marketing and advertising are used in ways that didn't even exist ten years ago, and how far we can or should utilise them to combat illness is undoubtably a very modern dilemma.

What shall I do?

There is a Chinese proverb that says 'It is better to light a single candle than curse the darkness', and this is an excellent motto to keep in mind; you undoubtably cope better with disaster if you do something rather than nothing. The problem is that the uncertainty and helplessness brought on by ill health can have a paralysing effect, making it much harder to know what exactly you should do 'for the best'. I think the answer is that it doesn't really matter *what* you do but being active rather than passive is going to help.

There will be many big things you can't control, but there are many small things that you can, and the very act of making a decision can help you to feel more in charge. You need to try and prevent yourself from feeling as if you are someone to whom things just happen and more like someone who has been authorised to act responsibly. Whatever you do is useful – don't worry about whether it's the right thing to do, just do something.

———

Chapter Sixteen

ONE DAY MORE

The Future

The patient's story?

A BOOK SUCH AS THIS could contain at least one chapter by the patient themselves. But only today, Alan says to me when I tell him (again) about this book, 'Well it's not as if I was in hospital for very long is it?', and almost falls off his chair when I remind him for the millionth time that he was away for almost a year. Not only can he not remember his year in hospital, he also can't really perceive the difference in himself before and after the illness. And when his neurologist or I ask him how he is, he'll answer in terms of how he feels at that precise moment. Asking him to write down his thoughts on what it's like to have a brain injury, what it's like to be Alan, always results in a blank sheet.

The mesmerising story of a month of autoimmune encephalitis, *Brain on Fire*, is a harrowing and vivid first-person account. Its author, Susannah Cahalan, has pieced together an extraordinary narrative from her own shattered memories and the accounts of her friends and family. But as she says, 'I'm an unreliable source.

No matter how much research I've done, the consciousness that defines me as a person wasn't present then.' Nevertheless, as well as being a superb writer, she has come through the experience with a whole level of self-awareness that is entirely missing from Alan. She was a 24-year-old woman and he a 67-year-old man, and of course, no two recoveries will be the same.

I hope that although Alan cannot help to write our story, reading it will empower him to know that he can move from being someone who needs help to someone who is helping. Passing on what you have learnt along the way can be part of the journey and the community of life-changing illness. And I wanted to tell the stories of both the patients and the carers, knitted together, because there isn't always as much of a difference as you might think between looking after others and looking after yourself. As Christie Watson points out, 'We are all nursed at some point in our lives. We are all nurses.'

We are family

Right from the start, I knew that if I hadn't had Izzy, Madeleine and Sam, the outcome of this horrible experience for both Alan and me would have been quite different and unutterably worse. It has made me beyond proud to see how they have coped with the shattering changes to their dad – and also the changes to their mum. The five of us have gone through this in our own ways but we also have gone through it together. I made the decision to tell as many people as possible; they made a different decision – to tell very few friends indeed. Izzy's boyfriend, Chris, stepped up to the mark in a way that belied his youth and showed him to be the compassionate and mature young man that he is. I believe it has made my children stronger, wiser, kinder – but the fact remains that losing the father you once had is astonishingly hard. Madeleine told me that when things were tough, she imagined Alan as he once was, standing next to her, encouraging her and saying, 'Well done Mads, you're doing really well, keep going', and I found this extremely moving.

A role in life

I hear Nadiya (*Bake Off*) Hussain talking on Radio 2, and she says that to start with she found it hard to be seen as a spokesperson for Muslim women, for working mums. She just wanted to be a baker. But now she wonders if maybe that's her role, her position in life, and embraces it. Maybe she's being the person she was supposed to be. It makes me wonder about that question of what we're 'supposed' to be and how it can change and surprise us. Maybe looking after Alan and now writing about illness is what I'm 'meant' to do?

My granddaughter Nancy, who is seven at the time, says to me one day, 'Granny, what's your job?' I pause. It's important to all of us to give her strong role models, to show her that a woman can do anything she chooses. Simon and Maddy both have jobs in the government, powerful jobs, weighty jobs. 'Well,' I say, 'my main job at the moment is looking after Grandpa.' I see her face fall slightly with the disappointment that it's not a bit more interesting and, to be honest, something falls inside me too. We need to change the narrative around caring – to show that it's a superpower, not an uninspiring humdrum task.

Change and growth

Post-traumatic growth is a term that was developed in the 1990s by Richard Tedeschi and Lawrence Calhoun to describe the concept of 'growth as a potential consequence of grappling with trauma'. They were interested in the people who had experienced a major crisis or disaster but had been able to use it to make positive, meaningful changes to their lives. This is a thought-provoking way of looking at what can happen after a serious illness, and it strikes a chord with me.

The two psychologists interviewed individuals who had survived many types of trauma: sometimes an illness such as blindness, a brain injury, cancer or paralysis, and sometimes an ordeal such as being held hostage or as a prisoner of war. Their clinical experience during these interviews suggested they were looking 'at a fundamental human experience from a fresh perspective'. Time and time again they heard the same thing. Although the losses that the participants and their families had experienced had caused them great sadness, they felt that, nevertheless, the experience had changed them for the better.

One of their many studies (1995) revealed that survivors reported benefits including 'an increased appreciation for life in general, more meaningful relationships, an increased sense of personal strength, changed priorities, and a richer existential and spiritual life'. An important aspect of their research is that 'post-traumatic growth is an ongoing process, not a static outcome'. This gives me great hope that we can move as a family to a place where we are not always thinking, 'Things were better before Alan was ill.'

Author Stephen Joseph also explored this concept in his book *What Doesn't Kill Us: The New Psychology of Posttraumatic Growth* and found that 'those who try to put their lives back together exactly as they were remain fractured and vulnerable. But those who accept the breakage and build themselves anew become more resilient and open to new ways of living.'

As I think about this, it is hard to come to terms with the difficult thought that Alan has not gained 'an increased sense of personal strength', but maybe I have. Perhaps his loss has led to my gain.

Pulling through

This is the end of my book, but it isn't the end of our story. As the years go by and events both good and bad fill them, the prism through which we view Alan's illness is forever tilting. I found it was all too tempting to assume that because one momentous thing had happened to our family, we had now had 'our share' of misfortune – but of course it doesn't work like that.

In 2020, the global pandemic ensured that the whole world had a taste of life-changing drama, and everyone started to focus on what it really meant to be seriously ill. That same year, within the space of a couple of months, my seemingly unstoppable mother was diagnosed with terminal cancer and passed away. For six weeks, Izzy, Madeleine and Sam did an amazing job of looking after Alan, while I went to Gloucestershire to help my dad to care for mum. Suddenly, the part of my brain that had previously been completely taken up with thinking about Alan's welfare was replaced with her, and the way I saw the world changed again.

Deciding what to call this book was tricky, partly because its story is ongoing. Should we use the ever-popular 'journey' word? I thought of Dr Audrey Daisley's phrase 'bounce forward'; we wanted something positive, but that sounded too sprightly, too light-hearted. Then I thought of our family and how we were buffeted by the choppy waters of Alan's illness, unsure of the way forward, tossing, turning and sometimes sinking. Gradually, I have realised that many others are in the same boat and, however stormy the sea, it is possible to pull through. With help.

If you were to meet Al tonight at a party, I think you'd enjoy chatting to him. He's a people person, good at small talk, he always was, and his brain has got quite good at not leading him into territories he can't navigate. Unless you asked him a direct question – Where are we? How did you get here? What day is it? – you maybe wouldn't even notice there was anything wrong. But tomorrow, he'd have no knowledge of either you or the party. I'm sometimes reminded of the famous Macbeth quote about life, the one that suggests it is 'a tale told by an idiot, full of sound and fury, signifying nothing'. However dramatic or momentous the occasion (a fireworks display, his own birthday, a 600-mile train journey through France, the birth of a grandchild, Christmas Day, a funeral), he won't remember it.

Memories are made of this

Almost three years to the day that Alan first went into hospital, I am standing outside my granddaughters' bedroom door, listening to Alan laughing with them. He is sitting on the floor with his back against their bunk bed, playing a daft game that I remember him playing with Izzy, Madeleine and Sam and which I know he played with Lucy and Simon when they were little, too. He pretends to glue their hands together and then professes extreme astonishment when it doesn't work and they can 'escape'. Esther is four and Tove is one, and they are giggling so hard they can't speak. Again and again, he does the same thing, and their peals of laughter get merrier and merrier. Then they get hiccups, which sets them all off into even louder jollity. The three long years when Alan wasn't capable of playing like this seem like a distant memory, and how glad I am that Alan is no longer 'ill Grandpa', he's now 'funny Grandpa'.

Yet at the same time, this perfect moment is hanging in its own twist in time. Minutes earlier, Alan couldn't remember where he was or what the girls' names were, and I know that by the next day, he won't be able to remember anything at all about this day.

Then it occurs to me that Esther and Tove are so young that they almost certainly won't remember it either. And just like Alan, neither girl is at all bothered by this, because none of them are aware of the limitations of their own recall. All three of them are suspended in a little world of here and now, a bubble of pure joy. And I'm certain that even if none of them can recollect it afterwards, the happiness will still be embedded inside them somewhere.

A MEDICAL JARGON BUSTER

Abdomen: tummy.

Acute: sudden and severe.

Anaesthesia: a medical way of relieving pain. A general anaesthetic means the patient will be unconscious; a local anaesthetic means the anaesthetist will just numb one part of the body.

Anaphylaxis: a severe and potentially life-threatening allergic reaction.

Aneurysm: a swelling in the wall of an artery.

Antibody: a blood protein produced by the body in response to a specific antigen.

Antigen: a substance that causes the immune system to produce antibodies against it. Examples include viruses, chemicals, pollen or bacteria.

Artery: a blood vessel carrying blood away from the heart to other parts of the body.

Atrial fibrillation: an irregular pulse.

Atrophy: the wasting away of part of the body.

Autoimmune response: when the body produces antibodies that react against the body's own tissues.

Canula: a thin tube inserted into a vein or an opening in the body to administer medication, drain off fluid or insert a surgical instrument.

Cardio: to do with the heart, as in the cardiology department.

Catheter: a small tube inserted through your urethra into your bladder in order to empty it.

Cerebral: to do with the brain.

Chemotherapy: the treatment of disease (especially cancer) using chemical substances.

Chronic: long term or persistent.

Cirrhosis: serious liver disease.

Cognitive: relating to thinking and reasoning.

Colon: part of the large intestine, leading down to the rectum.

Confabulation: a symptom of various brain disorders in which fabricated stories fill in any gaps in memory.

Coronary: to do with the heart.

CPR: cardiopulmonary resuscitation. This is an emergency procedure using chest compressions, often with artificial ventilation. It can save a person's life if their heart has stopped beating or they have stopped breathing.

Dialysis: the medical process of removing waste products and excess fluid from the body, which is necessary when the kidneys aren't working.

DNR: do not resuscitate. This means that a doctor is not required to resuscitate a patient if their heart or breathing stops. It is designed to prevent unnecessary suffering.

Dyspnoea: breathlessness.

-ectomy: a suffix meaning 'the removal of' a part of the body. For example, gastrectomy means taking out part of the stomach.

Embolism: where a piece of a blood clot, or something else, becomes stuck in a blood vessel.

Encephalitis: brain inflammation or swelling.

Endoscope: a long thin tube with a light and camera, which is put into the body through the mouth, bottom or a small incision. The procedure is called an endoscopy.

Epidural: an injection given in the back which provides anaesthesia that creates a band of numbness from the tummy button to the upper legs. Often used in childbirth.

Gastro: to do with the stomach.

Gynaecology: relating to medicine that deals with the functions specific to women and girls, especially those affecting the reproductive system.

Haematology: to do with blood.

Haemorrhage: very heavy bleeding.

HDU: high-dependency unit. This is for patients who still need a high level of treatment and nursing but less than in intensive care.

Hepatic: to do with the liver.

Hypertension: raised blood pressure.

Hypotension: low blood pressure.

ICU: intensive-care unit.

Inflamed: reddened, swollen, hot and often painful.

Intravenous (IV) drip: a small plastic tube that is inserted into a vein so that fluids or medicines can go directly into the bloodstream.

Invasive: any medical procedure in which a cut is made to the body or an instrument is inserted.

-itis: if this comes at the end of a word, it means inflammation; for example, appendicitis means an inflamed appendix.

Keyhole: a minimally invasive surgical method used to access the interior of the body through a very small incision.

Lymph: a colourless fluid containing white blood cells. A lymph node is a small gland in the lymphatic system.

Neurology: the study of disorders of the nervous system, which includes the brain, the spinal cord and nerves.

Nil by mouth: an instruction which means that you are not allowed to have any form of food, drink or medication through your mouth.

OB/GYN: a commonly used abbreviation used in female healthcare. OB is short for obstetrics or an obstetrician, a doctor who delivers babies. GYN is short for gynaecology.

Occlusion: the blockage of a blood vessel or hollow organ.

Oedema: swelling or fluid.

Oncology: the study and treatment of tumours.

Orthopaedic: dealing with the correction of deformities of bones or muscles.

-oscopy: a suffix meaning 'viewing of', so a colonoscopy means looking at the colon.

OT: occupational therapist, who helps patients improve their ability to do everyday tasks.

Paediatric: children's.

Palliative: care for the terminally (incurably) ill.

Pathology: the study of the causes and effects of disease.

Phlebotomy: opening a vein in order to withdraw blood.

Prostate: a gland within the male reproductive system, just below the bladder.

Psychosis: a condition affecting the way the brain processes information, causing a person to lose touch with reality. It is a symptom, not an illness in itself.

Pulmonary: to do with the lungs.

Radiotherapy: the treatment of disease (especially cancer) using X-rays or similar forms of radiation.

Remission: a (possibly temporary) decrease or disappearance of the severity of disease or pain.

Renal: to do with the kidneys.

Rheumatic: to do with joints, bones, cartilage, tendons, ligaments and muscles.

Sedation: a state of calm or sleep produced by a drug.

Sepsis: the immune system's overreaction to an infection or injury, which can lead to tissue damage, organ failure and death.

Stent: a very small tube inserted into a blood vessel to keep it open.

Sutures: stitches.

Tachycardia: a rapid heartbeat.

Thrombosis: a clot that develops in a blood vessel.

TIA: transient ischemic attack: a temporary blockage of blood to the brain, also known as a mini-stroke.

Urethra: the tube through which your urine empties out of your bladder.

Vascular: relating to vessels, especially those that carry blood.

Vessel: a channel such as a vein, in which a bodily fluid is carried.

Appendix Two

SOURCES OF HELP
AND SUPPORT

Age UK

www.ageuk.org.uk

This is a treasure trove of useful information on all sorts of things from benefits to knowing your employment rights.

Carers UK

www.carersuk.org

This is one of the most useful websites, with loads of helpful information, especially about financial and practical matters, and it should be better known. I think the issue is that people don't always think of themselves as 'carers'. But if you look after someone who is ill, whether they are your friend, child, parent or partner, you will find something useful here.

Citizens Advice

www.citizensadvice.org.uk

There is a lot of information on here that you might find particularly helpful if you have issues with housing, debt, employment, immigration or legal matters. It will also point you towards your nearest local Citizens Advice office where you can make an appointment to get free advice in person, on the phone or via an online chat.

Council info
www.gov.uk/find-local-council
Your local council is the place to find out about disabled parking permits, becoming a registered carer, accessing social care, family services, getting a reduction on your council tax and much more.

Department for Work and Pensions (DWP)
www.gov.uk/dwp
This is the government department responsible for the Personal Independence Payment (PIP), the Disability Living Allowance (DLA), the Attendance Allowance and other benefits. You will need to register on the website in order to access the right information for you.

Driving and DVLA
www.gov.uk/dvla
This is the place to find out about driving with medical conditions, Blue Badges and public transport if you're disabled, plus the rules on eyesight, toll concessions for disabilities and more.

Encephalitis Society
www.encephalitis.info
The Encephalitis Society raise awareness and provide support for both those who have had the illness and also their families. They are a worldwide organisation and aim to improve the quality of life of all people affected directly and indirectly by encephalitis by

being an invaluable source of information, as well as promoting and collaborating on research.

First aid

www.nhs.uk/conditions/first-aid

It was doing a first aid course at work that enabled me to save Alan's life, and I would strongly recommend that you read through the webpage above. There are also two good first aid apps created by the British Red Cross and St John Ambulance, which you can download on your phone for free.

Headway: The Brain Injury Association

www.headway.org.uk

Headway are a nationwide charity who aim to improve life after brain injury, whether it arises from an accident or an illness. A network of groups and branches across the UK provides a wide range of services, including rehabilitation programmes, carer support, social re-integration, community outreach and respite care, to survivors and families in their own communities. They also lobby for better support and resources to be made available to people affected by brain injury and work to raise awareness of the devastating effects that brain injury can have.

Integrated Neurological Services

www.ins.org.uk

Patients with neurological conditions have the lowest health-related quality of life of any long-term condition. INS use a holistic approach to deliver a range of integrated clinical services and social and emotional therapeutic support in West London. Their work reduces loneliness and depression, which contributes to improved wellbeing in patients and carers.

Macmillan Cancer Support

www.macmillan.org.uk

Macmillan Cancer Support are one of the largest British charities and provide specialist healthcare, information and financial support to people affected by cancer. They also look at the social, emotional and practical impact that cancer can have and campaign for better care.

NHS

www.nhs.uk

The NHS website is a huge resource. As well as containing a vast amount of information about pretty much every illness, it will enable you to find your nearest GP surgery, pharmacy, optician, dentist or hospital.

Which?

www.which.co.uk

You do not have to be a member to use this website, and there is lots of useful information about care, including NHS Continuing Healthcare (NHS CHC) and NHS-Funded Nursing Care (FNC). This is on the 'Services' page, and although it is entitled 'Later life care', there are lots of pointers towards care options that might be appropriate for you, whatever your age.

REFERENCES, BIBLIOGRAPHY AND FURTHER READING

Chapter Three: A Matter of Life and Death
The brink

Dylan, B. 'Don't Think Twice, It's All Right.' [Copyright: 1963 by Warner Bros. Inc.; renewed 1991 by Special Rider Music.]

Chapter Four: A Whole New World
Bad luck, good luck

NHS Confederation (2017) *'NHS statistics, facts and figures.'* 17 July. www.nhsconfed.org/resources/key-statistics-on-the-nhs

House of Commons Library (2019) *NHS Key Statistics: Briefing Paper 7281.* 31 May. http://researchbriefings.files.parliament.uk/documents/CBP-7281/CBP-7281.pdf

The World Bank (2017) 'World Bank and WHO: Half the world lacks access to essential health services.' 13 December. www.worldbank.org/en/news/press-release/2017/12/13/world-bank-who-half-world-lacks-access-to-essential-health-services-100-million-still-pushed-into-extreme-poverty-because-of-health-expenses

Coping with trauma

North Tees and Hartlepool NHS (2017) *Common Reactions to Traumatic Events.* www.nth.nhs.uk/content/uploads/2017/07/AE-1084-common-reactions-to-traumatic-events-july-2017.pdf

Assume nothing

Encephalitis Society (2019) *'Encephalitis explained: Autoimmune encephalitis.'* www.encephalitis.info/pages/category/autoimmune-encephalitis

Autoimmune Encephalitis Alliance (2016) *'FAQ: What is autoimmune encephalitis?'* http://aealliance.org/faq/#what-is-ae

Encephalitis: a quick guide

Encephalitis Society (2017) *'What is encephalitis?'* www.encephalitis.info/what-is-encephalitis

The problems of unusual illnesses

BBC Radio 2 (2020) 'Conversation with Dr Chris Smith.' *The Jeremy Vine Show.* 7 April.

Solomon, T. (2016) 'A Neurological Perspective.' In A. Easton *Life After Encephalitis: A Narrative Approach.* Routledge.

Wanting the world to know

Murrays Pharmacy (2018) 'Are crowdfunding sights promoting quack treatments for cancer?' 13 December. www.murrays.co.uk/blog/post/are-crowdfunding-sites-promoting-quack-treatments-for-cancer

The Guardian (2019) 'When survival is a popularity contest: The heartbreak of crowdfunding healthcare.' 20 May.

The Telegraph (2020) 'Can crowdfunding cancer treatment ever truly work?' 10 February.

CNN Health (2019) *'The average crowdfunding campaign for cancer care asks for $20,000 but only gets about $5,000.'* 9 September. www.edition.cnn.com/2019/09/09/health/medical-fundraising-unmet-goals-trnd/index.html

The BMJ (2018) 'Is cancer fundraising fuelling quackery?' 13 September. www.bmj.com/content/362/bmj.k3829

How doctors break bad news

Watson, C. (2018) *The Language of Kindness: A Nurse's Story*. Chatto and Windus.

Go your own way

Sontag, S. (2009) *Illness as Metaphor*. Penguin Books. (Original work published 1978.)

Ten (equally valid) ways to deal with illness

Thomas, D. (2016) 'Do Not Go Gentle into that Good Night.' In *The Collected Poems of Dylan Thomas*. Weidenfeld and Nicolson. (Original work published 1951.)

Winn, R. (2018) *The Salt Path*. Penguin.

Christopher and Dana Reeve Foundation (2020) *Today's Care, Tomorrow's Cure*. www.christopherreeve.org/research

Chapter Five: Hospital Hacks: The Practical Stuff

'The thing is, I really don't like hospitals'

Full Fact (2017) *'How many NHS employees are there?'* 1 June. http://fullfact.org/health/how-many-nhs-employees-are-there

A special relationship?

Kay, A. (2018) *This is Going to Hurt: Secret Diaries of a Junior Doctor.* Picador. (Reproduced with permission from Pan Macmillan through PLSclear.)

The Telegraph (2017) 'Hot wax was dripping down into his bladder – former doctor Adam Kay on revolting injuries and the future of the NHS.' 15 December. www.telegraph.co.uk/books/authors/hot-wax-dripping-bladder-former-doctor-adam-kay-revolting

An apple a day keeps the doctor away?

Department of Health and Social Care (2019) *'Hospital food review announced by government.'* 23 August. www.gov.uk/government/news/hospital-food-review-announced-by-government

World Health Organization (2020) *'Healthy diet fact sheet.'* www.who.int/news-room/fact-sheets/detail/healthy-diet

Nighty-night, sleep tight?

National Sleep Foundation (2020) *'Will a weighted blanket help you sleep better?'* www.sleep.org/articles/will-a-weighted-blanket-help-you-sleep-better

The Sleep Doctor (2019) *'Thinking of using a weighted blanket? Here's what you need to know.'* 23 April. www.thesleepdoctor.com/2019/04/23/thinking-of-using-a-weighted-blanket-heres-what-you-need-to-know

Medical News Today (2018) 'Is sleeping with socks on good for you?' March. www.medicalnewstoday.com/articles/321125

Walker, M. (2018) *Why We Sleep: The New Science of Sleep and Dreams.* Penguin.

BBC Science Focus (2020) *'Why does the smell of lavender help you sleep?'* www.sciencefocus.com/the-human-body/why-does-the-smell-of-lavender-help-you-sleep

The many tribulations of hospital parking

Express (2018) 'Scrap hospital parking charges: £2.50 could've saved my dad's life, says grieving daughter.' 15 June. www.express.co.uk/news/uk/974464/hospital-parking-fee-uk-scrap-charges

Mirror (2019) 'Mum spends life savings in hospital parking during daughter's cancer treatment.' 16 September. www.mirror.co.uk/news/uk-news/mum-spends-life-savings-hospital-20075891

The Guardian (2018) 'Hospitals making hundreds of millions from parking charges.' 27 December. www.theguardian.com/society/2018/dec/27/hospitals-making-hundreds-of-millions-from-parking-charges

BBC News (2018) *All hospital parking charges scrapped by the end of year.* 1 May. www.bbc.co.uk/news/uk-wales-south-east-wales-44069699

The Sunday Post (2013) 'Hospital car parking hell.' 8 September. www.sundaypost.com/news/uk-news/hospital-car-parking-hell

Adam Smith Institute (2017) *'Three cheers for hospital car parking charges.'* 16 November. www.adamsmith.org/blog/three-cheers-for-hospital-car-parking-charges

Parliament.co.uk (2019) *Hospital Car Parking Charges (Abolition) Bill 2017–19.* http://services.parliament.uk/Bills/2017-19/hospitalcarparkingchargesabolition.html

The hell of A&E

BBC News (2019) *'Boy slept on hospital floor due to lack of beds.'* 9 December. www.bbc.co.uk/news/uk-england-leeds-50713236

Chapter Six: How It All Works: The Mechanics of a Hospital
'What are you saying exactly, doctor?'

Sheather, J. (2019) *Is Medicine Still Good for Us?* Thames and Hudson.

Academy of Medical Royal Colleges (2018) *'Writing outpatient clinic*

letters to patients.' September. www.aomrc.org.uk/wp-content/
uploads/2018/09/Please_write_to_me_Guidance_010918.pdf

'They're doing some tests'

NHS Inform (2019) *'Tests and treatments.'* 9 July. www.nhsinform.scot/
tests-and-treatments

House of Commons Library (2019) *NHS Key Statistics: Briefing Paper 7281.*
31 May. http://researchbriefings.files.parliament.uk/documents/
CBP-7281/CBP-7281.pdf

Science Museum (2018) *'Brought to life, lab diagnostic machines.'* http://
broughttolife.sciencemuseum.org.uk/broughttolife/techniques/
labdiagnosticmachines

Blood is thicker than water

Oates, J. C. (1993) *I Lock My Door Upon Myself.* Ontario Review Press.

Nature (2017) 'Diagnosis: Frontiers in blood testing.' 27 September. www.
nature.com/articles/549S16a

Other tests and scans

NHS Inform (2019) *'Test and treatments: MRI scan.'* 9 July. www.
nhsinform.scot/tests-and-treatments/scans-and-x-rays/mri-scan

Brighton and Sussex NHS (2018) *Equipment, Devices and Procedures in
the Intensive Care Unit.* www.bsuh.nhs.uk/wp-content/uploads/
sites/5/2016/09/Equipment-devices-and-procedures-in-the-
Intensive-Care-Unit.pdf

Wikipedia (2020) *'Plasmapheresis.'* http://en.wikipedia.org/wiki/
plasmapheresis

Phones in hospitals

NHS.co.uk (2018) *'Common health questions: Use of mobile devices by*

patients in hospitals.' 23 July. www.nhsx.nhs.uk/covid-19-response/
data-and-information-governance/use-mobile-devices-patients-
hospitals-eg-phones-tablets-and-cameras

Information Government Alliance (2015) *The Use of Mobile Devices
in Hospital.* 15 October. https://digital.nhs.uk/data-and-
information/looking-after-information/data-security-and-
information-governance/codes-of-practice-for-handling-
information-in-health-and-care

Chapter Seven: All Hail the Hospital

A force for good

Watson, C. (2018) *The Language of Kindness: A Nurse's Story.* Chatto and
Windus.

A very short hospital history

Science Museum (n.d.) *'The history of hospitals.'* http://broughttolife.
sciencemuseum.org.uk/broughttolife/themes/hospitals

Journal of the Royal Society of Medicine (2006) 'A review of *A History
of Britain's Hospitals and the Background to the Medical, Nursing
and Allied Professions.'* www.ncbi.nlm.nih.gov/pmc/articles/
PMC1457754

Sheather, J. (2019) *Is Medicine Still Good for Us?* Thames and Hudson.

Cahalan, S. (2012) *Brain on Fire.* Penguin.

What I've learnt about the UK healthcare system

Gilbert, D. (2020) *The Patient Revolution: How We Can Heal the Healthcare
System.* Jessica Kingsley Publishers.

The phrase 'cradle to grave' was used in The Beveridge Report, published
in November 1942. It was drafted by the Liberal economist William
Beveridge and formed the basis for the post-war reforms known

as the Welfare State, which included the creation of the National Health Service.

Patients Know Best (2020) *'Your health in your hands.'* www.patientsknowbest.com

Coe, J. (2018) *Middle England.* Vintage Press.

Hendry, D. (2001) 'Poem for a Hospital Wall.' In *Borderers.* Peterloo Poets. (Reproduced with kind permission from Diana Hendry.)

Chapter Eight: It's a Family Affair: Talking and Listening to Children, Siblings and Parents

Children and hospitals

Morpurgo, M. (2007) *Cool!* HarperCollins Children's Books.

The power of youth

Care Quality Commission (2018) *NHS Children and Young People's Patient Experience Survey.* www.cqc.org.uk/sites/default/files/20191119_cyp18_statisticalrelease.pdf

The Guardian (2018) 'Children in care homes.' 12 November. www.theguardian.com/society/2018/nov/12/children-care-homes-residents-feel-more-human

Age UK (2018) *'How care homes and nurseries are coming together for good.'* 26 April. www.ageukmobility.co.uk/mobility-news/article/intergenerational-care

Building family resilience

Daisley, A., Tams, R. and Kischka, U. (2009) *Head Injury: The Facts.* Oxford University Press.

Walsh, F. (2006) *Strengthening Family Resilience* (2nd edition). New York: The Guilford Press.

Dr Daisley's strategies

Talk given by Dr Audrey Daisley, Consultant Clinical Neuropsychologist, Royal Society of Medicine, London, July 2017. (Reproduced with kind permission from Audrey Daisley.) There is lots of useful information by Dr Audrey Daisley about supporting families with brain injuries on the BrainLine website: www.brainline.org/author/audrey-daisley-dclinpsych-cpsych.

When kids become carers

Your Support Service (2018) *'Revealed: 800,000 young carers in England.'* www.yss.org.uk/news/new-bbc-news-figures-reveal-800000-young-carers-in-england

Chapter Nine: You've Got a Friend in Me: Assembling an Army

You don't bring me flowers

NICS Well (2009) 'You don't bring me flowers anymore.' www.nicswell.co.uk/health-news/you-dont-bring-me-flowers-anymore

Perfect presents for hospital patients

MIT News (2015) 'Recalling happier memories can reverse depression.' 17 June. http://news.mit.edu/2015/recalling-happier-memories-reverse-depression-0617

Chapter Ten: Reasons to be Cheerful: How to be Happy in Hard Times

The power of laughter

BBC Radio 2 (2018) 'What makes us human? An essay by Marian Keyes.' *The Jeremy Vine Show.* 5 June.

Always look on the bright side

Alcott, L. M. (2018) *Little Women.* Wordsworth Editions. (Original work published 1968.)

Coolidge, S. (2017) *What Katy Did.* Virago. (Original work published 1872.)

Burnett, F. H. (2018) *The Secret Garden.* Arcturus Press. (Original work published 1911.)

Ingalls Wilder, L. (2014) *Little House on the Prairie.* Egmont. (Original work published 1932.)

Spyri, J. (2018) *Heidi.* Puffin. (Original work published 1881.)

Green, J. (2013) *The Fault in Our Stars.* Penguin.

Downham, J. (2012) *Before I Die.* David Fickling Books.

Porter, E. H. (2018) *Pollyanna.* Puffin Classics. (Original work published 1913.)

Turn that frown upside down

The London Economic (2019) 'Always look on the bright side of life: Optimists really do live longer.' 26 August. www.thelondoneconomic. com/lifestyle/health/always-look-on-the-bright-side-of-life-optimists-really-do-live-longer-157787

Sontag, S. (2009) *Illness as Metaphor.* Penguin Books. (Original work published 1978.)

Ehrenreich, B. (2009) *Bright-Sided: How the Relentless Promotion of Positive Thinking Has Undermined America.* Metropolitan Books.

Researchgate.net (2013) *'Always look on the bright side of life: Cancer and positive thinking.'* March. www.researchgate.net/ publication/258154387_Always_look_on_the_bright_side_of_life_ Cancer_and_positive_thinking

And he drove the fastest milk cart in the west

Fotopoulou, A., Conway, M. A. and Solms, M. (2007) 'Confabulation: Motivated reality monitoring.' *Neuropsychologia 45* (10) 2180–2190.

Be more sisu

BBC (2018) *'Sisu: The Finnish art of inner strength.'* 7 May. www.bbc.com/worklife/article/20180502-sisu-the-finnish-art-of-inner-strength

Reasons to be cheerful

Independent (1998) 'Ian Dury: Great sense of tumour.' 17 August. www.independent.co.uk/arts-entertainment/interview-ian-dury-great-sense-of-tumour-1172226.html

Jankel, C. J., Payne, D. S. and Dury, I. R. *Reasons to Be Cheerful Part 3.* Peermusic Publishing, Warner Chappell Music, Inc.

Jankel, C. J. and Dury, I. R. *Spasticus (Autisticus).* Emi Longitude Music Co.

Accentuate the positive

O'Donnell, L. (2014) *Cancer is My Teacher.* Independently published. www.cancerismyteacher.com

Stupid Cancer Stories (2020) *'The Survivor Thriver Series 10: Toni Crews.'* http://blog.stupidcancer.org/the-survivor-thriver-series-10-toni-crews-d248a82e9fd5

Only connect

Independent Age (2019) *'Campaign to end loneliness, the threat to health.'* www.campaigntoendloneliness.org/threat-to-health

Holt-Lunstad, J., Smith, T. B., Baker, M., Harris, T. and Stephenson, D. (2015) 'Loneliness and social isolation as risk factors for mortality: A meta-analytic review.' *Perspectives on Psychological Science*

10 (2) 227–237. www.researchgate.net/publication/273910450_
Loneliness_and_Social_Isolation_as_Risk_Factors_for_
Mortality_A_Meta-Analytic_Review

A friendly face

BBC News (2018) *'Many hospital patients get no visitors.'* 11 September.
www.bbc.co.uk/news/health-49633721

Chapter Eleven: Crazy for You: The Mental Health of the Patient and the Carer

O, let me not be mad

Walker, J., Burke, K., Wanat, M., Fisher, R., Fielding, J., Mulick, A.,
Puntis, S., Sharpe, J., Degli, M., Harriss, E., Frost, C. and Sharpe,
M. (2018) 'The prevalence of depression in general hospital
inpatients: A systematic review.' *University of Oxford.* http://ora.
ox.ac.uk/objects/uuid:7ea8e6a5-3540-42b2-b51e-678a63633b78/
download_file?file_format=pdf&safe_filename=Walker_2018_
Psych%2BMed_Prevalence%2Bof%2BDepression.pdf&type_of_
work=Journal+article

DiMatteo, M. R., Lepper, H. S. and Croghan, T. W. (2000) 'Depression
is a risk factor for noncompliance with medical treatment:
Meta-analysis of the effects of anxiety and depression on patient
adherence.' *Archives of Internal Medicine 160* 2101–2107.

Journal of Neuroscience Nursing (1981) 'Brain injury and the family.'
https://journals.lww.com/jnnonline/Citation/1981/08000/
Brain_Injury_and_the_Family.2.aspx

Mental Health Foundation (2020) *Long Term Conditions and
Mental Health.* www.mentalhealth.org.uk/a-to-z/l/long-term-
physical-conditions-and-mental-health

The lunatics have taken over the asylum
Kesey, K. (1962) *One Flew Over the Cuckoo's Nest*. Penguin Classics.
BBC News (2014) *'Obituary for PD James.'* 27 November. www.bbc.co.uk/news/uk-10787952

A short timeline of mental health care in Britain
The National Archives (2020) *'Lunatic asylums, psychiatric hospitals and mental health.'* www.nationalarchives.gov.uk/help-with-your-research/research-guides/mental-health
Science Museum (2020) *'Exploring the history of medicine.'* http://broughttolife.sciencemuseum.org.uk/broughttolife/techniques/bethlemroyalhospital
Independent (2012) 'The demise of the asylum and the rise of care in the community.' 26 November. www.independent.co.uk/life-style/health-and-families/health-news/the-demise-of-the-asylum-and-the-rise-of-care-in-the-community-8352927.html
BBC Health (2017) 'Steep rise in A&E psychiatric patients.' 10 January. www.bbc.co.uk/news/health-38576368
Cahalan, S. (2012) *Brain on Fire*. Penguin.
Watson, C. (2018) *The Language of Kindness: A Nurse's Story*. Chatto and Windus.

All in the mind?
BBC News (2014) *'Scans chart how quickly babies' brains grow.'* 12 August. www.bbc.co.uk/news/health-28740495

'She's not usually like this'
Murdoch, A. (2017) *Bed 12*. Hikari Press.
Headway: The Brain Injury Association (2019) *'The emotional effects of brain injury.'* www.headway.org.uk/about-brain-injury/individuals/effects-of-brain-injury/emotional-effects

Losing your mind

ScienceDirect (2012) *'Unusual psychiatric syndromes.'* www.sciencedirect.
    com/topics/neuroscience/capgras-delusion

Cahalan, S. (2012) *Brain on Fire*. Penguin.

Dark thoughts acknowledged

Talk given by Dr Audrey Daisley, Consultant Clinical Neuropsychologist,
    Royal Society of Medicine, London, July 2017. There is lots of useful
    information by Dr Audrey Daisley about supporting families with
    brain injuries on the BrainLine website: www.brainline.org/author/
    audrey-daisley-dclinpsych-cpsych.

Caring for the carers

Carers UK (2020) *'Looking after your health, stress and depression.'* www.
    carersuk.org/help-and-advice/health/looking-after-your-health/
    stress-and-depression

Healing harmonies

Rolling Stone Magazine (1986) 'Billy Joel: The Rolling Stone Interview.'
    11 December.

BBC News (2019) *'Music "calms nerves before surgery" as well as sedative.'*
    19 July. www.bbc.co.uk/news/health-49033435

Chapter Twelve: Using the Outside to Help the Inside: The Healing Power of Nature

Nature's balm

English Heritage Magazine (2017) 'How to garden like a mediaeval monk.'
    7 April.

A room with a view

Science (1984) 'A view through a window may influence recovery from surgery.' 27 April. www.researchgate.net/publication/17043718_ View_Through_a_Window_May_Influence_Recovery_from_ Surgery

Academia (1999) *The Health Benefits of Gardens in Hospitals.* www.academia.edu/8672345/Health_Benefits_of_Gardens_ in_Hospitals._Roger_S._Ulrich_Ph.D

Blowing away the dark humours

Clarke, R. (2020) *Dear Life: A Doctor's Story of Love and Loss.* Little Brown.

BBC Radio 2 (2020) 'Rachel Clarke interview.' *The Jeremy Vine Show.* 29 January.

Jarman, D. (1992) *Modern Nature: The Journals of Derek Jarman.* Vintage Classics.

Dennis Potter in an interview with Melvyn Bragg on 15 March 1994. Broadcast by Channel 4 on 5 April 1994.

The seeds of regrowth

BBC 3 (2017) *Judi Dench: My Passion for Trees.*

Wohlleben, P. (2017) *The Hidden Life of Trees: What They Feel, How They Communicate: Discoveries from a Secret World.* William Collins.

Shinrin-yoku (forest bathing)

Association of Nature and Forest Therapy Guides and Programs (2020) www.natureandforesttherapy.org

Association of Nature and Forest Therapy Guides and Programs (2019) *'Science agrees: Nature is good for you.' A collection of journalism and research on the health benefits of nature and forest therapy.* www. natureandforesttherapy.org/about/science

School of Agriculture and Food Science, University College Dublin (2015) *The Benefits of Group Walking in Forests for People with Significant Mental Ill-Health.* December.

Green prescriptions

British Medical Association (2019) *'Nature's remedy: Doctors in Shetland give green prescriptions.'* 20 July. www.bma.org.uk/news/2019/july/natures-remedy-doctors-in-shetland-give-green-prescriptions

The Telegraph (2016) 'Do you need a green prescription?' 17 September. www.telegraph.co.uk/health-fitness/body/do-you-need-a-green-prescription

The circle of life

The Telegraph (2019) 'Gardening can do what medicine only "tries to mimic" for mental health.' 24 February. www.telegraph.co.uk/news/2019/02/24/gardening-can-do-medicine-tries-mimic-mental-health-monty-don

Chapter Thirteen: Recovery: Normal Service will not be Resumed

'You must be so happy he's home!'

Marriott, H. (2014) *The Selfish Pig's Guide to Caring.* Piatkus Press. (Original work published 2003.)

Adjusting and adapting

Hattenstone, S. (2016) 'Foreword.' In A. Easton *Life After Encephalitis: A Narrative Approach.* Routledge.

The long and winding road

Daisley, A., Tams, R. and Kischka, U. (2009) *Head Injury: The Facts.* Oxford University Press.

Walsh, F. (2006) *Strengthening Family Resilience* (2nd edition). New York: The Guilford Press.

Rehabilitation, recuperation and restoration

Encephalitis Society, Jackson, H. and Morton, N. (2002) *'Rehabilitation after encephalitis.'* (Updated March 2017.) www.encephalitis.info/rehabilitation-after-encephalitis

You have a choice

BBC Radio Gloucestershire (2019) *Fighting Cancer with Fashion.* 2 December.

Look after yourself

Carers UK (2020) *'Facts and figures about carers and the people they care for.'* www.carersuk.org/news-and-campaigns/press-releases/facts-and-figures

NHS (2020) *'Conditions: High blood pressure.'* www.nhs.uk/conditions/high-blood-pressure-hypertension

Chatterjee, R. (2019) *Feel Better in 5: Your Daily Plan to Feel Great for Life.* Penguin.

Chapter Fourteen: Help! Getting the Practical Support You Need

Respite care

Alzheimer's Research UK (2018) *'Dementia statistics: The impact on carers.'* 14 August. www.dementiastatistics.org/statistics/impact-on-carers

Which? (2019) *'Day care centres: We explain how to arrange day care, the perfect way to give you a few hours' break from caring on a regular basis.'* 26 April. www.which.co.uk/later-life-care/carers-and-caring/respite-care/day-care-centres-amty8ou1pott

Encephalitis Society (2020) *'Rehabilitation after encephalitis.'* www.encephalitis.info/rehabilitation-after-encephalitis

Keep taking the tablets

Age UK (2019) *More Harm Than Good: Why More Isn't Always Better with Older People's Medicines.* June 2019. www.ageuk.org.uk/globalassets/age-uk/documents/reports-and-publications/reports-and-briefings/health--wellbeing/medication/190819_more_harm_than_good.pdf

Council tax reduction

MoneySavingExpert (2017) *'Revealed: Councils overcharging 10,000s who are severely mentally impaired.'* 29 September. www.moneysavingexpert.com/news/2017/09/revealed-councils-overcharging-10000s-who-are-severely-mentally-impaired

MoneySavingExpert (2019) *'How to claim the severely mentally impaired council tax discount.'* 22 October. www.moneysavingexpert.com/reclaim/severe-mental-impairment-dementia-council-tax-rebate

Charitable help

The Book Trade Charity: www.btbs.org

Encephalitis Society: www.encephalitis.info

Integrated Neurological Services: www.ins.org.uk

Headway: The Brain Injury Association: www.headway.org.uk

Homelink: www.homelinkdaycare.co.uk

Chapter Fifteen: The Big Questions

I need answers

Kundera, M. (2020) *The Unbearable Lightness of Being*. Faber and Faber. (Original work published 1984.)

I should be so lucky?

The Guardian (2017) 'The secret to success? Believe in luck.' 11 April.

BBC News (2011) *'Why do we believe in luck?'* 6 April. www.bbc.co.uk/news/magazine-12934253

The Guardian (2016) 'The psychology of luck: How superstition can help you win.' 25 July. www.theguardian.com/lifeandstyle/2016/jul/25/psychology-donald-trump-win-luck-superstition

Halla, M., Liu, C. and Liu, J. (2019) *The Effect of Superstition on Health*. Institute of Labor Economics. http://ftp.iza.org/dp12066.pdf

Medical News Today (2019) 'How do superstitions affect our psychology and wellbeing?' 13 September. www.medicalnewstoday.com/articles/326330

The New York Times (2006) 'In science based medicine, where does luck fit in?' 19 September. www.nytimes.com/2006/09/19/health/19essa.html

Ackerman, C. (2020) 'What is Positive Mindset: 89 Ways to Achieve a Positive Mental Attitude.' 13 October. www.positivepsychology.com/positive-mindset

Does 'what doesn't kill you make you stronger'?

BBC News (2019) *'Tree of the Year 2019.'* www.bbc.co.uk/news/uk-england-49632776

Do the drugs work?

The Daily Telegraph (2019) 'The new anti-vaxxers: Why fake cancer cures are on the rise.' 23 June, p.19.

The Guardian (2019) 'Measles cases up 300% worldwide in 2019, says WHO.' 15 April, p.20.

Shall I tell you a story?

Irani, S. (2016) 'A Neurological Perspective.' In A. Easton *Life After Encephalitis: A Narrative Approach*. Routledge Press.

Sacks, O. (2011) *The Man Who Mistook His Wife for a Hat*. Picador Classic. (Original work published 1985.)

Clarke, R. (2020) *Dear Life: A Doctor's Story of Love and Loss*. UK publisher: Little Brown. US publisher: Thomas Dunne Books. (Reproduced with kind permission from Little, Brown Book Group in the UK and Aitken Alexander on behalf of Thomas Dunne Books in the US.)

Barnes, J. (2012) *The Sense of an Ending*. Vintage.

Easton, A. (2016) *Life After Encephalitis: A Narrative Approach*. Routledge Press.

Has 'He' got the whole world in his hands?

RTÉ One (2015) 'The meaning of life.' Stephen Fry in an interview with Gay Byrne. 1 February.

Independent.ie (2017) 'Irish girl who survived Manchester terror bombing that killed 22 people had guardian angel watching her.' 23 May.

Are doctors a higher species?

The Guardian (2019) 'Real NHS doctors too busy to care about patients.' 16 October. www.theguardian.com/society/2019/oct/16/real-nhs-doctors-too-busy-to-care-about-patients-says-bodies-creator

The Telegraph (2017) '"Hot wax was dripping down into his bladder" – former doctor Adam Kay on "revolting" injuries and the future

of the NHS.' 5 December. www.telegraph.co.uk/books/authors/
hot-wax-dripping-bladder-former-doctor-adam-kay-revolting

Kay, A. (2018) *This is Going to Hurt: Secret Diaries of a Junior Doctor.*
Picador. (Reproduced with permission from Pan Macmillan
through PLSclear.)

Does life matter?

Dickens, C. (2013) *Dr Marigold.* A Word to the Wise. (Original work
published 1865.)

Watson, C. (2018) *The Language of Kindness: A Nurse's Story.* Chatto and
Windus.

Gawande, A. (2015) *Being Mortal: Illness, Medicine and What Matters in
the End.* Profile Books.

How real are memories?

The Guardian (2019) 'My wife lost her memory while giving birth.' 5
October.

Barnes, J. (2012) *The Sense of an Ending.* Vintage.

Is life fair?

Los Angeles Times (2008) 'Fairness, idealism and other atrocities.' 4 May.
www.latimes.com/archives/la-xpm-2008-may-04-op-orourke4-
story.html

Should illness be marketed?

Independent (2019) 'Breast cancer survivor criticises "fluffy" pink charity
ribbons.' 7 November. www.independent.co.uk/life-style/women/
breast-cancer-audrey-birt-survivor-pink-ribbons-cancer-pretty-
pink-a9189036.html

Easton, A. (2016) *Life After Encephalitis: A Narrative Approach.* Routledge
Press.

BreastCancerNow.Org (2017) *'The history of the pink ribbon.'* 10 October. breastcancernow.org/about-us/news-personal-stories/history-pink-ribbon#history-pink-ribbon

Birt, A. (2019) *'Pink ribbons, black dogs and equity.'* 10 November. audreybirt.blogspot.com/2019/11/pink-ribbons-black-dogs-and-equity.html

Daily Mail, The (2019) 'The Pink Ribbon rebellion.' 7 November. www.dailymail.co.uk/news/article-7662767/The-pink-ribbon-rebellion-Two-prominent-breast-cancer-survivors-share-opposing-views.html

Independent (1994) 'Inquiry into guide dog charity's spare £160 million pounds.' 6 October. www.independent.co.uk/news/inquiry-into-guide-dog-charitys-spare-pounds-160m-1443347.html

MarieCurie.org (2018) *'What does the yellow flower daffodil pin mean?'* October. www.mariecurie.org.uk/blog/daffodil-pin-meaning/183716

Chapter Sixteen: One Day More: The Future

The patient's story?

Cahalan, S. (2012) *Brain on Fire*. Penguin.

Watson, C. (2018) *The Language of Kindness: A Nurse's Story*. Chatto and Windus.

We are family

Easton, A. (2016) *Life After Encephalitis: A Narrative Approach*. Routledge Press.

Change and growth

Tedeschi, R. G. and Calhoun, L. G. (1995) *Trauma & Transformation: Growing in the Aftermath of Suffering*. Sage Publications. https://psycnet.apa.org/record/1995-98741-000

Tedeschi, R., Park, C. and Calhoun, L. (1998) *Posttraumatic Growth: Positive Changes in the Aftermath of Crisis.* Routledge.

Tedeschi, R., Shakespeare-Finch, J., Taku, K. and Calhoun, L. (2018) *Posttraumatic Growth: Theory, Research, and Applications.* Routledge.

Joseph, S. (2013) *What Doesn't Kill Us: The New Psychology of Posttraumatic Growth.* Basic Books.

Sheather, J. (2019) *Is Medicine Still Good for Us?* Thames and Hudson.

INDEX